WEST COUNTRY DOCTOR is a warm and compelling account of the tribulations and triumphs of a Somerset doctor working in a farming and mining community.

Based on life in a real practice, Dr Lane's recall of patients and people is both funny and tragic, heartwarming and perceptive.

'Kenneth Lane's DIARY OF A MEDICAL NOBODY was a wonderful invocation of 1930s medicine, as nostalgic as a forgotten whiff of friar's balsam or iodoform. I enjoyed it immensely'
Richard Gordon, author of DOCTOR IN THE HOUSE

Also by Kenneth Lane
DIARY OF A MEDICAL NOBODY
and published by Corgi Books

West Country Doctor

Kenneth Lane

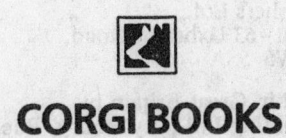

CORGI BOOKS

WEST COUNTRY DOCTOR

A CORGI BOOK 0 552 12465 6

Originally published in Great Britain by Severn House
Publishers Ltd.

PRINTING HISTORY

Severn House edition published 1984
Corgi edition published 1985

This book is set in 10/11 English Times

Corgi Books are published by
Transworld Publishers Ltd.,
Century House, 61–63 Uxbridge Road,
Ealing, London W5 5SA

Made and printed in Great Britain by
Hunt Barnard Printing Ltd., Aylesbury, Bucks.

To avoid any possibility of embarrassment to friends or relatives of those who were my patients in the nineteen forties, circumstances as well as names have been changed in many of my stories. My aim has been to entertain and perhaps occasionally to inform.

1

The year was 1938 and I believed at the time that it must be the heyday, the golden age of our lives. Jessica and I had been married eight years and during that time I had metamorphosed from a hesitant youth just out of medical school to an established partner in one of the oldest and best practices in the country. If this sounds as though I am boasting — well of course I am.

Almost nine years earlier, in the summer of 1929, we had presented ourselves to Dr John Symonds, senior partner of the practice in Melbrook, Somerset. We were twenty-three years old and engaged. John Symonds appeared to us as elderly at forty-eight and formidable. Needing another junior partner, he had written to Guy's Hospital requesting that a series of suitable young doctors should be sent down for his approval.

'We always have Guy's men, Lane,' he had said with such solid pride and confidence that I had been prepared to become the lowest form of life in such a practice if only I could get my foot in the door.

The hospital record of any doctor applying for the job was regarded as enough to guarantee his medical ability, but his character and personality and even more that of his wife or fiancée were of paramount importance. Each couple was interviewed and entertained over a weekend or two while their suitability was assessed. We had several rivals. I have written elsewhere of the kind fortune that induced Jessica to wear a hat which the senior partner's wife found so completely irresistible that our future was virtually assured after that first lunch party at the Symonds. Of course it wasn't only the hat, it was the face of the girl under it that decided matters. She was clearly a young woman who would be able to charm the most difficult of patients out of their sulks and would have half the male population calling at our house to see her. Then in due course they would naturally become my patients. Any reasonable young doctor with such an asset at his disposal was bound to succeed. As it turned out things had indeed gone well for us.

On Saturday June 18th 1938 I met 'Dragon' at Bath station. We had long ago given up asking why she was called Dragon. It was her name, like Sally or Jane, and had no more significance. She was solidly built, barely five feet tall and nearly as wide, her deep voice could be gentle and her ample bosom could lull the most restless baby into a quiet sleep.

She was so much in demand as a resident midwife that it was said you had to book her before conception and not after. 'Well dear,' I heard her say to one disappointed expectant mother, 'you must book me first and have your petting party afterwards.' Not an altogether practical suggestion but it appealed to Dragon's quiet sense of self-esteem.

As we drove up the long hill south of Bath she asked, 'A boy this time Doc?'

'I don't mind a bit,' I replied. 'I rather like the pattern of product we've established so far.'

'Jessica would like a boy, I'm sure,' she said.

'Possibly. But she'll be happy enough with either.'

Our third baby was due on June 20th but for some reason labour was delayed. This was embarrassing because Dragon had been booked for the regulation four weeks and delayed labour meant she would have to leave for her next case before the baby was four weeks old. So we did our best to get things started.

All the routine techniques of uterine stimulation available to us at that time were tried and failed. First there was the drive over the bumpy road to Tyning. This was a track that might well trouble the commander of a centurion tank but it had no effect. When this failed, Jessica was told by Dragon to polish the nursery floor. She was so flexible and mobile that this gave her no bother and had no effect either. I remember watching her on her hands and knees, polishing away and smiling up at me from time to time. Eventually Dragon relaxed to a routine of afternoon rests and evening snoozes and we settled down to wait.

On June 29th, Jan — our eldest — remembers Jessica coming into the nursery and saying, 'I think this would be a very nice day to have a baby,' which she did without fuss or trouble later that day.

Tom Wyburn, my partner, was in attendance and I sat on the stairs waiting for the first cries of the baby. It must have been ten minutes after the first sturdy bellow that Tom came out on to the landing drying his hands. 'Another girl,' he told me. He just saved himself from saying 'I'm afraid' and I knew he thought we should be disappointed. There is supposed to be something not quite decent about a father who prefers daughters. For myself I was delighted. If we had had a dozen little Jessicas I should have been a dozen times delighted so long as we could afford all they needed.

And so Catharine arrived.

In those days the mother stayed strictly in bed for fourteen days, doing exercises to strengthen the pelvic floor, feeding and playing with the baby. It was splendid treatment for both mother and child. Visitors were received at fixed and limited times and the room was filled with flowers.

Three months later Neville Chamberlain was making his famous 'peace in our time' speech at London Airport. It has become fashionable to condemn him, but those of us who were preparing our minds for war ought to admit that for a time we were profoundly relieved.

As the months passed, Jan aged seven, Pat aged four and Catharine aged a few months became the centre of our lives. In spite of the gathering clouds of war there was plenty to laugh at. At quite an early age Pat became the doctor in the nursery and Jan — three years older — the matron: a very proper distribution of authority when you consider the importance of matrons. I remember Pat on one occasion getting to the telephone before anyone else and on being told someone wanted me replying, 'He's very busy. He's eating his dinner.'

My home life had a considerable effect on my attitude to patients. For a long time, for instance, I was unsympathetic towards marital problems because in my own life they didn't exist. 'We only know what we have experienced' is a truth I learned very slowly.

Many of the tales I have to tell of those busy years of my life in family practice consist of my education in the art of understanding people. I learnt much from Jessica. Her knowledge was intuitive, mine was painfully acquired.

The marriage of Mark and Valencia Dubcross was outwardly a bitterly unhappy one, but the dramatic end to my relationship with this couple makes the story worth telling.

Valencia, in her forties, still bore signs that she had once been good-looking. Her figure had become fuller but gave evidence that it had once been pretty well perfect. Physically her health was excellent yet for many years she was one of my 'chronics'. Ever since I had known her she had complained of every conceivable symptom, of agonising pains all over her body, of tinglings, of itchings, of giddiness and of states of exhaustion such as no one had been expected to put up with since the world began.

It is difficult to imagine the strange nature of these complaints. Were they real? Imaginary? Or merely a means of demanding help from the doctor, the healer? I still don't know the answer but of one thing I am sure. It is even more difficult to forecast the reaction of the spouse to these complainers.

A typical consultation with Valencia Dubcross would go something like this. 'I've got that terrifying pain in my hips again and right up my back to my neck.'

'How long have you had it this time?'

'Five days and nights. I haven't shut my eyes. I don't expect you can do anything about it, but I thought I would come on the off-chance that there is something new.'

I had previously had her spine Xrayed, had her blood tested and had made full examinations. She had seen several consultants, none of whom had found any evidence of physical disease.

I had asked long ago about stresses, anxieties and tensions but the answer was always the same. 'I am not a nervous person. There is something radically wrong with me.'

When I asked about her marriage I was put firmly in my place. 'I'll not discuss my private affairs with anyone. There's too much talk of sex these days and it does no one any good.'

Seizing a chance to talk to Mark one day I had learned little more. He admitted that his wife 'did nag him rather' and that he had accordingly found it difficult to feel any sexual attraction for her. In fact sex had ceased to be a part of their marriage some years ago.

So I was reduced to giving Valencia Dubcross bottles of old-fashioned bromide and nux vomica which for some reason she demanded from time to time. She was firmly registered as one of my failures.

Then she developed signs of genuine physical disease and investigation showed that she had developed a cancer of the stomach.

A surgeon operated but a year later signs of secondary growth made her outlook virtually hopeless. After another spell in hospital she was sent home to find what comfort she could in her remaining months. It was impossible to keep the truth from her and the knowledge that she had cancer did nothing to reduce the level of her complaints. By this time she was convinced that she had had the cancer for many years and that I and the consultants who had seen her had grossly neglected her and were directly responsible for her hopeless condition. It was useless to tell her that the pathologist had reported that the cancer removed at operation had been an early one. Doctors would always back each other up, she said, but she knew better.

At first everyone, nurses and neighbours, were full of sympathy but gradually her constant complaining began to wear them down. No one was outwardly impatient. Who could be with a victim of cancer? But attitudes changed, sympathy was forced, good will was taxed to its limit.

11

Mark, the husband, suffered almost as much as the wife. Some thought more. After a couple of months he was in a bad way. He seemed one of those men who are born to suffer and long ago a look of resignation had settled on his face. As time went on, loss of sleep and constant nagging left their mark on him in the form of pale patches round his mouth and nose and deepening lines about his eyes.

After each of my visits to the wife I came away telling myself how sorry I was for the husband and had to keep reminding myself who was the invalid. The conversation usually went something like this.

'Well and how are you, Valencia?'

'You know quite well how I am, Doctor. I am dying and things are not being made easy for me.' Her look asked for an enquiry that duly came. 'My husband is being appallingly difficult and so selfish. You'd think he would be willing to put me first just for these few weeks, but not him.'

'You mean you need more help? More domestic help? Mark is still working. I suppose he has to if he's going to keep his job.'

'When I may die any day?'

'I don't think it's as bad as that. You haven't lost any more weight and there's no sign that things are getting worse.'

'Last night I couldn't sleep and he snored for hours on end. Then about four o'clock when I did drop off for a few minutes, he started sighing and groaning and saying he couldn't sleep.' She spoke as though Mark had been guilty of inexpressible crimes including rape, murder and robbery with violence.

'I expect he was tired from his day's work. He cooks when he comes home, doesn't he?'

'He only has to put it in the oven.'

'What did you have for supper yesterday for instance?'

'A little soup and some fish pie.'

'And who made that?'

'He did make that and a nice mess he made of it.'

'How much could you do yourself? Could you do a little in the kitchen for instance?'

'I don't think even you know how bad I feel. You don't know the half of it.'

I knew I was being unsympathetic. 'Tell me, is there something else worrying you?'

'Of course there is.' Anger and hatred seemed to be fighting for dominance in her expression. 'He's only waiting for me to die and he'll marry that woman over the road.'

'Who do you mean?'

'The merry widow they call her. Mrs Breeze.'

'Surely you can't think that. Mark has always been so devoted to you.'

'Devoted to her you mean. The sooner I'm dead and gone the better.'

I asked the district nurse whether she thought Mrs Dubcross was exaggerating her symptoms. It seemed a hard thing to say of a woman dying of cancer, but I felt sure at this stage that a little more activity would be good for her. The nurse was emphatic. 'That's putting it mildly,' she said. 'It's that poor husband I feel sorry for.'

One day I asked Mark how he was coping with a strenuous job and a sick wife at the same time. 'I've always been too hard on her,' he said. 'I used to think she made a fuss over nothing but now she's got this terrible thing I feel I want to make it up to her. I'd do anything I could to make her comfortable — anything.' The absence of any hint of complaint over his lot was impressive.

The weeks and months wore on. The patient lost some weight but otherwise there was not much change. Mark looked all in, haggard, pale and wretched. Two years after the operation, when she had lasted longer than expected, she began to go downhill and was needing morphia for her pain but she still looked as though she would last another few weeks.

One scene stays in my memory. I was standing on one side of her bed and Mark on the other. She was looking ill but the morphia was keeping her free from pain and quite relaxed. She glanced from one to the other of us with something malicious in her expression. 'There you are, both of you,' she said. 'You've both failed me completely from beginning to end.'

My first reaction was anger which I had to suppress. I

had done my best but Mark's behaviour had been almost saintly. For years he had spent all his energies on making her as comfortable as possible. I glanced at him but his face was void of all expression. He had probably, I thought, grown immune over the years to an unending succession of cruel stabs.

I puzzled over the seemingly unrelieved evil of her disposition but later another idea struck me. She had been obsessed by one thought. The men she had to deal with had to be failures. She had to emasculate us in her own estimation. We had to be impotent. Was this the deep-seated cause of all her behaviour? And could psycho-analysis have elicited the reason for it?

I didn't know but such theorising was soon forgotten. A day or two later, quite suddenly, she developed diarrhoea and vomiting, collapsed and died.

To say I was puzzled is an understatement. Something had intervened. Some sort of food poisoning? Poison. The word struck me like a blow. Was it possible? The thought shocked me. This was something that happened to other people, not to my patients.

The vomiting and diarrhoea had started at about ten in the morning. It was Sunday and Mark was at home, but he didn't send for me until teatime by which time she was on the point of death. What was more, every trace of vomit and excreta had been meticulously cleared away.

I asked him why he hadn't sent earlier and he said that after the first half-hour his wife had made no complaint at all and he didn't want to trouble me. I asked why he hadn't at least kept the vomit. This was a routine precaution known to every first-aider. He told me he had wanted to keep the place clean and fresh.

Then came the problem of the death certificate. It was to be an ordinary burial, not a cremation, so only one death certificate was needed. She had suffered from cancer and her case was hopeless. This much was well documented. But I had expected her to live another month or two and something else had intervened to cause her sudden death. Was it possible that Mark Dubcross, a mild kindly man, patiently devoted to a very trying wife, could

14

have been tormented beyond endurance?

How well did I really know him? Was it possible that under that gentle exterior were hidden depths of hatred for a woman who had made his life a misery for years? But this was complete nonsense and I knew beyond any possibility of doubt that Mark had not hated his wife and would never have raised a finger to hurt her.

There was however another possibility. Could he have been so distressed by her suffering that he had decided to give her an overdose of drugs to put an end to her misery? She had been on morphia and night sedation and neither of these would cause vomiting and diarrhoea. Could he have given her some other poison in the hope of saving her from a month or two of painful dying? It was impossible to be sure but could he have cleared away all the evidence of the final cause of death in complete innocence?

Any mention of gastroenteritis on the death certificate would automatically call for a coroner's enquiry. Was I imagining things and could I really put the poor man to all the misery and suspicion that would inevitably follow? He had been sorely tried for years and the last months must have been hell for him. A full enquiry, public suspicion and endless delays were the best that could be expected if I mentioned gastroenteritis. If I was certain in my own mind that the sole cause of death was cancer of the stomach and the diarrhoea was only terminal, I had every right to sign the certificate accordingly. But was I certain?

It was one of those cases you couldn't discuss with anyone. If a question was even raised the answer was obvious: it should be reported to the coroner. Yet the mere seeking of his opinion would cast doubts on the integrity of a man who was probably completely innocent.

I tried hard to find a simple explanation for the terminal symptoms. Perhaps there had been secondary growth irritating the intestine: that was too far-fetched. Perhaps there had been some degree of kidney failure: that wouldn't do either.

The horrible question of Mark's innocence insisted on presenting itself to me over and over again. Then I remembered Valencia complaining that Mark was only waiting for her to die when he would marry the 'widow over the road'. All that evening I pondered and worried and at last I decided to call on Mark again, hoping that the interview would help me to make up my mind.

Careful not to give any hint of my suspicions, I began by asking him to give me an account of his wife's activities, such as they were, during the past week, and every detail of her diet. He answered carefully with every evidence of complete frankness. There was nothing to suggest food poisoning, she had eaten nothing that he hadn't had too. Then I looked at her remaining drugs and these appeared to be in order.

'She had no other medicines besides what I gave her? No patent medicines?'

'Nothing you didn't give her. Rather a blessing she died as she did, I've been thinking. Saved her a lot of suffering.'

'That's true but it's difficult to understand what happened — what caused the diarrhoea and sickness.'

He shook his head and sat back very calmly seeming to look into the distance. Did this indicate honesty or should it make me suspicious? Surely one should expect some sign of grief over the death of a wife, even if he hadn't loved her for years.

I went home still in doubt.

I couldn't sleep and in the early hours Jessica and I talked the affair over agan. 'If you are in any doubt you ought to report it to the coroner,' she said. 'Ring him up and ask him. You've done that before.'

'If I do he's bound to demand an inquest. If one expresses the slightest doubt the answer is obvious.'

'Well, you are in dousbt.'

'I don't really doubt Mark Dubcross and I'd be causing him a lot of unnecessary misery and worry when he's already had as much as he can take.'

'Didn't you tell me once that his wife had said he was only waiting for her to die before he married some widow?'

'I've been thinking that too. It was only her spite of course.'

16

'Are you sure? You are just trying to protect the man from a little worry at the expense of your own peace of mind.'

'Suppose he was trying to save her from suffering?'

Jessica was silent for a while then came out with some of her usual simple practical wisdom. 'That's not for you to decide, is it? That's the coroner's job.'

'O.K., you're right. I'll report it to the coroner.'

I did so with a heavy heart first thing next morning. A post-mortem was ordered and an inquest would follow if necessary.

At lunch-time there was a call from Mark's neighbour. Mark had been taken suddenly ill with vomiting and diarrhoea. My relief was enormous and I drove cheerfully up to see him before I began my lunch. His symptoms were similar to those of his wife but he was far less acutely ill in himself. It was obvious now that some sort of infection was the cause of the whole trouble. All my fears had been groundless.

Post-mortem revealed widespread growth but no cause for the diarrhoea which was presumed to be infective. They failed to isolate the organism concerned but there was no evidence of poison. Mark recovered in a day or two but in the wife's weak state the infection had proved too much for her. There was no inquest and that concluded the affair.

And Mark didn't marry the widow over the road.

2

General Practice is truly family practice and involvement in family affairs is one of its joys, and sometimes one of its greatest sorrows.

One morning in the spring of 1939 a young woman named Penelope Daker sat opposite me in the surgery. She was eighteen years old, not beautiful but with a pleasantly serious face. She was neatly dressed in a jacket and skirt, an attractive blouse and — joy of those days — a small hat worn a little on one side, not jauntily but enough to be pleasing.

I was glad to see her because the surgery that day had been a dull affair. There was still a great deal of winter infection about and treatment could only be palliative. Penicillin was not yet on the market and sulphonamide was used only for serious infections.

Penny had a small lump on the back of her wrist — a pleasant sight at that particular moment because the diagnosis was obvious and the treatment easy. She had a ganglion — a collection of fluid on one of the tendon sheaths — which could easily be dispersed. The classical treatment was to strike the ganglion a lively blow with the family bible, and no doubt in days gone by the holiness of the book would be credited with the instant disappearance of the lump.

I told Penny what it was and struck it a moderate blow with *French's Differential Diagnosis*, a book I kept mainly for this piece of therapy. The lump disappeared and she beamed with pleasure. At least I had done something useful and straightforward with my morning.

I expected her to express rapid thanks and leave me to

carry on with my other patients, but she seemed reluctant to go. She sat there as though she wanted to say something else and I waited. 'I wanted to talk to you about something else really,' she said. 'I don't know if you can do anything to help but I just wondered. You know Father very well and he likes you. Well, he and I are sort of at loggerheads at the moment because I want to ask a boy home and he doesn't think he's suitable — whatever suitable means.' She stopped a moment and took a deep breath. 'You see, he's a Barnado boy and he works on another farm on the Mendips.'

'You mean as a labourer? What makes him unsuitable, being a Barnado boy or being a labourer?'

'Both. Pa says he's only a farm worker and I've no business to go on seeing him. Also as he's a Barnado boy, we don't know anything about his family or background and that simply won't do. Then of course he says I'm too young, I'm only infatuated, I'm getting myself talked about and so on and so on. He won't listen to me and he makes me so *mad*.'

Her father had a large farm a few miles out of Melbrook and a hard tennis court where I sometimes played on Saturday afternoons. He was a man of self-assurance and strong character. His success was built on integrity and a rigid sense of justice. He was at the same time an absolute dictator in his own family.

'Are you serious about the boy?'

She shook her head as though no one would ever understand and spoke slowly. 'I love him. And I know I shall always love him. He's different from anyone else I've ever met.'

'I see. What do you think I can do about it?'

'Well if you come and play tennis one Saturday, could you talk to Father? I think he'd take notice of you.'

'Tell me more about the boy. How old is he?'

'He's twenty. There's another thing. He's in the Territorials so if there's a war he'll be called up in spite of doing farm work. I'm afraid he'll become involved in the war and we shall get separated. I'm terribly happy about him because I know he'll do well and in time we shall get

19

married. But I do want Father and Mother to meet him. I wouldn't worry if there wasn't a war coming.' The words rushed out of her as though they had been pent up for a long time. 'I couldn't bear him to go away for ages without anyone knowing we are engaged.'

'Engaged? It's as serious as that? Have you got a ring?'

'Not a proper one yet.' She pulled out a cheap little ring fixed to a chain round her neck. 'I daren't wear it on my finger so I keep it like this.'

'What's his name and where does he work?'

'Michael Manson.' She told me the farm he worked on. 'You saw him once. You vaccinated him.'

I tried to remember. 'I don't really know anything about him, but when I see your father I'll try and put in a word somehow. I doubt whether it will do any good. Your father isn't easily persuaded.'

So I was left with the unenviable task of 'putting in a word' for a young man I had only seen once for about two minutes. I ought to have told Penny I couldn't do anything to help her but I was convinced she was in love and I was an incurable romantic.

One Saturday afternoon I managed to sit out a set with Pa Daker and after a lot of hesitation I said, 'Penny came to see me the other day. She's worried, isn't she?'

He looked at me hard and I could feel the blue eyes boring through my head. 'Has she been talking to you about this boy of hers?'

'She wants you to meet him before you condemn him.'

'I haven't condemned the boy. I merely told her that a farm labourer wouldn't be able to give her the sort of home she's used to. Can you imagine young Penny settling down to thirty shillings a week and a tied cottage?'

'No, I can't, but if you are going to break the affair up I would have thought the best way is to let her see him in her own surroundings. The infatuation might fade smartly away then.'

'I shan't allow any such thing. It would be asking for trouble.'

'The problem is to get Penny to see the affair as you do without hurting her too much.'

'You think it's that serious?'

I felt sure the ecstatic happiness I had caught a glimpse of did mean something. 'There's a war coming,' I said, 'and he's in the Territorials so he'll be in the army. This could easily glamorise him. There won't be much class distinction in the army these days. Suppose he got a commission, you'd separate her more easily from a farm labourer than from a good-looking young officer.'

One Saturday afternoon some weeks later, I met Michael Manson at the Dakers'. So the stern father had agreed to see the boy. He was well-built, six feet tall with a good face. He spoke with a Somerset accent — but so did Mr Daker.

I was curious to know how the affair was progressing and what had made Penny's father relent. When I had an opportunity I asked how he liked him.

'You can't help liking him in a way,' he said. 'He looks well, has good manners — though I don't know where he gets them from. And of course Penny's mad about him.'

'I'm glad you are meeting him anyway.'

'It was you persuaded me to and it was a mistake. Far better not to have encouraged it.'

I gathered that he was favourably but reluctantly impressed, but the problem remained that a farm labourer was no fit partner for his daughter.

Curiosity made me attempt an assessment of young Michael's character and one showery day when we were driven indoors I had a chance to talk to him. He didn't play tennis and when he was present, neither did Penny.

'How long have you been working on the farm?' I asked him.

'Nearly three years now.'

'Quite a good life?'

'Yes, it's a good life.'

'What made you join the Territorials?'

'When I read about the Nazis I knew there was bound to be a war sooner or later and I wanted to be in it, that was all.'

'What about the conflict with farm work?'

'Now I'm in the terriers I'll be safe for the army. If there was a choice the army came first.'

'And after the war? Any ideas for a career?'

21

'I like farming. But after the war may be a long way off.'

'If there hadn't been a war would you have stuck to farming?'

'I think so. I've got no money. At least not that sort of money. But I should have worked my way up to farm management somehow.'

I liked his determination and his confidence. 'I always imagined farming was something of a closed community,' I said. 'Difficult to get into.'

'Not too difficult nowadays.'

He was articulate and had definite opinions. Even more important, he had the courtesy that comes of being truly aware of other people. I was thirty-three at that time and he was twenty, yet I felt he was the same age as I was. There was some solid personality there. I seized every opportunity to talk to him during the next few months. Perhaps we met three or four times. I gathered that he and Penny met about once a week, went to dances together and wrote to each other nearly every day.

One day he said, 'I've got a book by Thomas Hardy. *Far from the Madding Crowd*. I've read it three times.' He smiled half-apologetically. 'There's a character named Gabriel Oak — a solid man who made his way to the top on a farm. I still think it can be done.'

'He married the boss's daughter — or rather the owner of the farm.'

He smiled and said nothing. I liked the way he didn't feel obliged to continue a conversation if he had nothing to say.

'You like Thomas Hardy?'

'Yes, I've read all his books two or three times over.'

'A good choice. He's one of the few classics of the century. Any other favourites?'

'Not like Hardy.'

'What do you really like about him?'

'I've wondered myself.' He spoke slowly. 'It's partly the atmosphere. Partly that the books are about a really peaceful time. And partly that I like his words, the way he writes.' He stopped for a moment and I sympathised with

22

anyone trying to put into words what they liked about an author. 'There's one time,' he went on, 'when he describes Oak sitting out in the fields at night watching the constellations of stars go slowly past the world. And it made him feel the world was small, like a ship sailing through space. I like that.'

It always surprises me that casual conversation can produce such a definite opinion of character. There is a liking or disliking of course, but quite apart from that there is very soon a conviction about integrity, sincerity and trustworthiness. The safety of our neolithic ancestors must often have depended on instinctive judgements of this sort. I liked this boy. I was convinced he would make a career for himself and would be a suitable husband for Penny.

I took the opportunity to express my opinion to Mr Daker. 'That boy will make a career alright,' I said. 'I would be willing to bet he'll do very well.'

'You might be right,' he replied, but wouldn't volunteer anything more encouraging.

All through the months of that spring and summer we knew that war was inevitable. My partner, Tom Wyburn, was a major in the Territorials and would be called up before hostilities actually began. We calculated that as it had taken us four years to defeat Germany in 1914 it would doubtless take us another four years to defeat her now. Therefore, we planned, Wyburn should serve the first two years in the R.A.M.C. and I would serve the next two years. However naïve this sounds, it was amazing how it worked out — except that the war lasted six years, so Tom served two of them and I the other four.

In the middle of August, war had still not been declared and it was decided that I should take my holiday, so on August 16th we set out, Jessica and I and the three children, for North Wales where we had spent every summer holiday since we were married. The mountains, the sea, picnics, swimming and walking were to give us one more glorious fortnight before the war changed everyone's lives.

We arrived in Snowdonia in the early evening of a

perfect summer day. In Wales it was possible to delude yourself that the war was a nightmare that would disappear with the daylight tomorrow. Everything was normal — the yachts on the Straits of Anglesey, the singing and the mountains that had seen wars come and go many many times before.

When the children had gone to bed we stood, Jessica and I, looking down at the Straits where the moonlight was so strong that you could see the reflection of the church spire opposite in the still water. The weather would be perfect and for a time we could forget Hitler and his armies.

Next morning there was a telephone call from Tom Wyburn. His voice was measured and calm as usual. 'I've just been told that I have to stand by for call-up at four hours notice,' he told me, and waited for the news to sink in. 'I'm afraid this means that you will have to come back.'

'But we've only just got here,' I said. 'You mean you want us to come — when?'

'Today, I'm afraid.'

'I can get back in seven hours if the call-up really comes. Why not wait for it? It might be weeks before it happens.'

'It won't do, Lane. I couldn't leave this end of the practice without anyone to hold it for seven hours.'

'I don't see why not. One of the others would cope with any emergencies.'

'And suppose the war starts as we expect by massive bombing and probably gas attacks. You might never be able to make the journey at all.'

The picture that presented itself was horrific but it was one that had been in our minds for a long time. I knew the holiday was doomed. 'O.K.', I said grimly. 'We'll come back today.'

'Thank you.' The voice was almost caressing and for once it made me angry. How urgent was it really?

The world seemed to grow darker. Jessica stood beside me as I put down the telephone and for a moment we clung to each other.

The children were bitterly disappointed. On the journey

home they rebelled in fury at the cruelty of fate. To have smelt the sea and the tang of boats, to have glimpsed those lovely mountains and looked with excitement at the haze that promised a perfect day and then to have your heart's desire snatched away from you was enough to madden a choir of angels. And our children were not angels.

For a time we did our best to cheer them up but it was a hopeless task. After several hours of the journey home, Jessica began to read to them but for once this was no good. The distant look in their eyes when I managed to glance at them told clearly enough that their minds were far away on the seashore, they were messing about in boats or following us up mountain tracks that must inevitably lead to heaven at the top. It was a sad journey and one they still remember as the first traumatic experience of their lives.

We had a few days holiday at home and might just as well have stayed in Wales. It was nearly a fortnight before Wyburn was actually called up.

We listened to Neville Chamberlain's solemn broadcast on September 3rd and we were as ready as we could be for the holocaust. I was responsible for the first aid arrangements for the area and every night a party of four St John Ambulance men slept in their clothes in the surgery waiting-room with the ambulance outside. Gradually everyone got used to the phoney war but the first aid parties were unflagging in their alertness.

Sergeant Paragon of the St John Ambulance Brigade was responsible for the arrangements and he, thank heaven, was a character. Without a few rugged individuals the affairs of civil defence would be intolerably boring because in Somerset, far enough away from Bath and Bristol, there was likely to be far more waiting about than activity.

During the early months of the war I visited the first aid team every evening and on one occasion I must have been later than usual. The men were lying down in various stages of undress. Henry Paragon was in his shirt and pants but he promptly stood up, put on his steel helmet and shouted 'Stand up men! Let's have a bit of discipline.'

The sight of Paragon, trouserless in a long white shirt with his helmet on, calling for discipline, somehow stays in the memory. I told them to relax and asked if there was anything they wanted.

'A vew noice young wummen 'ouldn't do us no 'arm, Darcter,' said one of the men.

'Hampson!' shouted Paragon.

'Ver company I der mean.' Hampson looked quizzically at his leader.

'They're in short supply at the moment,' I told him. 'Shall I ask Miss Woodruff if she has any suggestions?' Miss Woodruff, our secretary dispenser, was the very efficient commandant of the Red Cross. The job suited her better than tamely putting up bottles of medicine.

'Per'aps ef you did racommend it zir,' grinned Hampson.

'That'll do, Hampson!' shouted Paragon again.

'Arry's too old yer zee, Darcter.'

'That's all you know.' Paragon was outraged now and I left them, no doubt arguing more freely without my presence.

The sense of comradeship that marked the war years was already growing into an invisible shield that did much to protect our morale from the disastrous news that followed like hammer blows for the next two or three years.

Just before Christmas that year I met Penny Daker in the town. There had been no tennis since the war began and I hadn't seen her or her family. She was full of excitement. 'Two pieces of good news,' she said. 'Mich has gone to O.C.T.U. which means he'll have his commission by February. Isn't it wonderful?'

I was very pleased, partly because I felt a small share in her happiness and partly because it was good to have my opinion of Michael reinforced.

'And look at this!' Penny showed me the ring on her engagement finger, the same one that she had worn so long round her neck. She wouldn't have any other, she said, even if Michael could afford it. She was so obviously happy that her joy helped to light up my day. 'And to think,' she went on, 'that if it hadn't been for that lump on my hand, it wouldn't have happened!'

This of course was nonsense, but I had realised long ago that in our job it is permissible to accept gratitude when you don't deserve it, because it makes up for some of the grumbles you don't deserve either.

I didn't see Penny again until the following June when we were all completely absorbed in the problem of the evacuation of Dunkirk. Churchill's solemn warnings filled the air and those perfect spring days followed when thousands of tiny boats were ploughing to and fro over the Channel. We seemed to hold our breaths in fear and hope. Young Michael Manson was among the troops in Flanders and no one knew what had happened to him. Penny, like thousands of others, waited in a fever of anxiety. At last we heard that he was in England, though one of the last to be evacuated. I think I was almost as relieved as Penny. He came to the Dakers' on leave and one day I met him in the town.

He had matured since I had last seen him a year earlier and was looking remarkably fit and handsome in his battledress with one pip on the shoulder. We shook hands and I asked him how things had been.

'Not bad,' he said.

'I hear you were in the perimeter defences with a good chance of being left behind.'

'They got all my little lot away. I came back in a fishing smack from Margate on the last day.'

'Tired?'

'None the worse.'

Penny clung to his arm and her pride was touching to see.

They were married that autumn and Jessica and I were asked to the wedding. It was a quiet affair but I always remember it because of the happiness that radiated from young Penny. Before they left she came up to me and kissed me. 'That's just to say thank you,' she said.

'What was the kiss for?' Jessica asked me later.

'I'm supposed to have persuaded Pa Daker that Michael was a good prospect as a husband,' I said. 'It's a sort of legend with Penny so I'll just let it ride!'

Four years later in June 1944, when I was in Naples, I

heard that Michael had been killed in Normandy. I could only imagine Penny's grief but in later years I came to know its depth. Intense joy is usually balanced sooner or later by intense pain. Yet if one had the chance to avoid the one at the expense of the other, who would do so?

3

During the first year of the war I was looking after some five thousand patients scattered over about a hundred square miles of Somerset. This sounds a vast area but when expressed as a radius of six or seven miles from my home it is less impressive. All the same I was very busy. Country patients who were ill had no means of transport to the surgery because petrol was rationed and buses a rarity, so on some days in the winter I did between thirty and forty visits as well as spending four hours or so in consultations in the surgery.

It was against this background that I had to decide whether to take on the major surgical operations of the practice which had previously been done by Tom Wyburn. Hospital beds in the city hospital were being kept as empty as possible that autumn in preparation for war casualties, and this presupposed that we should do our own surgery using the beds in the cottage hospital. I had made no clear decision about this when one November evening I had a call to see a miner's daughter with appendicitis.

I had been an assistant house surgeon at Guy's ten years before but although I had assisted Wyburn regularly I had done no abdominal surgery since. In those days you felt you had to do your share of whatever work came your way so long as you were reasonably competent to do it. And often enough the only person to judge your competence was yourself!

I decided to operate and looking back I am amazed at the sheer audacity of the young fellow I then was. At about eleven o'clock that evening we had the girl on the operating table. Dr Anderson, the Radwell partner who

29

had replaced Dr Symonds, was a competent anaesthetist and I had no anxiety on that score. If I had been able to foresee the events of the next hour I should have rushed to the telephone to shout for help, or better still have transferred the girl to the city hospital. As it was I stood calm and confident, waiting for the anaesthetist to give the word for me to begin.

I made the small incision generally used for straightforward cases of uncomplicated appendicitis. This was my first mistake. The way to hell is paved with small incisions, as many a good surgeon has taught. On the other hand, if successful the scar would be almost negligible, and this mattered in the case of an attractive young woman. I opened the abdomen. Alright so far. Nothing could go wrong and I expected the appendix to appear at once. Then for an agonising minute I couldn't find it.

This was absurd, I told myself, as my pulse began to rise in spite of my determination to remain absolutely calm. Then, moving the small intestines in the area where the appendix ought to be, I felt a small mass. Or was it a small mass? It was the size of a hen's egg. Was I dealing with something much more sinister than an acute appendix? The thoughts that occur to you under these conditions have to be experienced to be believed. Had the girl got a cancer of the bowel? Or an intestinal obstruction? Or Krohn's Disease? What had I let myself in for?

I brought the lump to the surface and found it was a mass of adhesions binding some coils of small intestine together and enclosing what was almost certainly an inflamed appendix. So my diagnosis was right. All I had to do was to remove the appendix. But the appendix was a mile away under loops of intestine which must not on any account be damaged. If I accidentally cut into the intestine, peritonitis would very likely follow. And we had no penicillin in those days to help in ironing out our mistakes.

The adhesions were of long standing, indicating a previous attack of appendicitis. I had asked the girl about these and she had denied any such possibility. Evidently she and her mother had forgotten some particularly bad 'tummy ache' of the past.

The problem was to undo the adhesions so as to be able to remove the appendix without damaging it. Cutting into the appendix would spread the infection all over the abdomen. With infinite care I set about unravelling the tangle, gently pulling the coils apart and cutting slowly through the adhesions. I had to be far more careful than an experienced surgeon would need to be. If you can imagine yourself in a race against the clock, unravelling a tangled skein of rope on a ledge of a precipice with the knowledge that if you took too long you would be overwhelmed by an avalanche, you will get some idea of my feelings. It must have taken me over half an hour to separate the appendix but at last it stood up, red and swollen but intact as far as I could see, and ready for removal.

Jim Anderson's quiet Scottish voice roused me from a world that seemed to have engulfed me for years. 'How's it going?' he asked.

'Alright now. Shan't be long.'

The rest was easy and I had a purse string suture in place and the appendix out in a few minutes. I stitched up the abdomen in the usual layers and thankfully pulled off my gloves while Matron applied the dressings.

'Thank you Matron,' I said politely.

'A nasty case for you, Doctor.' Did I imagine she was giving me a hint that I ought not to take on such a responsibility or was she being genuinely sympathetic?

Already a vague sense of guilt was disturbing me. The operation had taken over an hour and I was soaked with sweat. I went home and for the first time for years I couldn't sleep. I had suffered from the illusion that the best way to help the war effort was to work harder, but this was short-sighted. There had been no need to tackle an abdominal emergency when I was so completely out of practice. Nowadays when all surgery is done by specialists it would be unthinkable. I thought over the problem during the night and finally decided that if a surgeon was available he should be asked to do our surgery, even if he was working a hundred and sixty-eight hours a week.

I talked to one of the surgeons in the city hospital and described what I had had to do. He told me what I wanted to hear, that it was impossible to look after five thousand patients and have the worry of major surgery as well. He would willingly perform any surgery we had and would come out to the cottage hospital to do it if there was no available bed in the city. I was enormously relieved.

The girl made a perfect recovery and was discharged in about ten days, full of gratitude, but I felt no temptation to repeat my surgical adventure.

The most embarrassing thing about the whole affair was the gratitude of the parents. The girl's father came to see me, bringing a hare as a present. 'We'm prarper thankful to yeou, zir. And the girl she'm that proud of the mark of the operation. Ef ever me or my vamily needs a operation — which we'm not lookin' vor moind — we 'opes you'll do 'un.'

I couldn't understand why my reputation as a surgeon should blossom so suddenly on the basis of one appendicectomy, but I discovered the reason later. One of the junior nurses who had been present in the operating theatre that night had described the extreme technical difficulty of it and how masterly had been my achievement! I still blush to think about it. What an experienced surgeon would have done in twenty minutes had taken me three times as long. Never was bubble reputation more scantily based.

The fact is that junior nurses and medical students sometimes find a glamorous reflected glory in some very ordinary piece of surgery by describing it as something remarkable. The surgeon must be brilliant and the difficulties well nigh insuperable, then the glory in which they share is enhanced. The only credit I can claim is that I carefully drew back from the abyss that might have engulfed me. I was duly thankful for the good fortune that all had gone so well.

Hannah Woodruff, of course, saw through the undeserved praise. 'So Peterdown has got a new surgical, star, has it?' she said to me. 'Do we call you Mr Lane now or is Doctor still good enough?'

I mumbled something about our having had rather a party, but was never much at ease with our secretary dispenser.

During the winter of 1939/40 the fear of gas attacks

receded. The war hardly existed for us and I became completely immersed in the routine undramatic work of general practice. It was in the spring of 1940 that trivialities fell suddenly into proper perspective and I had my first real contact with the war. I was called urgently to a plane crash two miles away. An Anson training aircraft had crashed into a narrow wood between two meadows. I hurried over to Radwell and ran across a field to the spot. Some firemen had got there first and were opening a way into the fuselage. I clambered up into the wreckage and was greeted by a strong smell of petrol.

'I shouldn't strike a match if I was you, Doctor.' The advice from one of the firemen would have sounded comic in any other situation. Inside the Anson were six bodies of young men, all between the ages of twenty and twenty-four. My only task was to make sure they were all dead.

I examined the six young bodies who would have been laughing and joking together only half an hour earlier. They were all dead. Later I met and talked with the mother of one of them. He was her only son.

This was when the war actually began for me, but even this tragedy faded in the memory a few days later because Germany invaded Belgium and the phoney war was over.

It was at this time that we had a phone call one day from Harwich. It was from Jessica's French friend Thérèse Chesnais who had got away from Amsterdam with her two children and landed in England. She was in an advanced state of pregnancy and had nothing more than a suitcase full of clothes.

I remember hearing Jessica say 'You must come here of course. Get a train from London to Bath and we'll meet you there.'

This we did and for the next fifteen months the family shared our home. They were shattered when France fell but we were, of course, completely absorbed in the problem of the evacuation of Dunkirk.

I did my best to take no notice of the constant irritation caused by my relationship with Hannah Woodruff, but as time went on needless annoyance added to very long hours of work made me consider finding someone to replace her.

Her obsequious behaviour to the rich in contrast to her contempt for the poorer patients had infuriated me from the first day I joined the practice, but it was difficult to tell someone twice your age how to behave. Recapitulation of the countless occasions when she had angered me would make them sound trivial. Hannah Woodruff and I rubbed each other up the wrong way and in my ninety-hour weeks I needed help, not hindrance. The last straw came towards the end of 1940.

One afternoon I was late for surgery which was due to begin at four o'clock. I had been attending an elderly primip, a woman of thirty-five who was having her first baby, and hadn't wanted to leave her in the final stages of labour. In fact I had promised that I would deliver her myself. I did so and all went well but I didn't get away from the house until about half-past four.

I found the surgery packed with patients. We had no appointment system at that time and it was a case of first come first served. I was greeted by a very irritable Hannah Woodruff. 'Mrs Bold has been waiting since four o'clock,' she said. 'She's in your room.'

One is usually good-tempered after the successful conclusion of a maternity case and I murmured that I was sorry to be late. Mrs Bold was one of Wyburn's cases and a friend of Hannah Woodruff's. She was a large woman and as cross as Miss Woodruff at being kept waiting. I apologised for the delay and asked what was the trouble.

'It's my back,' she said. 'I've had agonies of pain down here,' she indicated her lower spine, 'for three months and I can't put up with it any longer.'

I had expected some emergency as she had been put ahead of all the other patients. If she had arrived at four o'clock she was out of turn because people always began to appear at half-past three, sometimes earlier. However it seemed a bit harsh to turn her out of the room now, and so long as the consultation could be fairly brief I would see her first. But as every doctor who has been more than about ten minutes in general practice knows, low back pain is almost as much of a trial to the doctor as to the patient.

I decided after a five-minute examination that this was an orthopaedic backache and an Xray was the first necessity. I wrote a note for this to be done at the cottage hospital and suggested pain relievers in the meantime. With thirty patients waiting to see me this should have been the end of the consultation.

'You don't know what is causing the pain then?' Mrs Bold demanded.

'Not yet, no. As soon as I've seen the Xray I'll decide on the next step.'

'So you are giving me tablets for a pain although you don't know what's causing it?'

'That's right, yes.'

'Well I'm not prepared to take pain killers until I know what's the matter.'

'Just as you like,' I said. 'We'll get the Xray done straight away — tomorrow probably. Telephone the hospital and Matron will give you an appointment. Then you must see me again.'

'But I have a right to know what it might be and what you expect to find in the Xray.' She sat firmly in her chair. 'Could it be cancer?'

At last I understood. She was terrified of cancer and frightened even to admit her fears. 'No,' I said 'it's definitely not cancer.'

'How do you know?'

'I have examined you and there is no sign of cancer.'

Still she sat there as though determined to spend the evening in my presence, but she was being seen out of turn while many others who should have been seen first were still waiting. I stood up. 'What time did you arrive this afternoon?'

'At four o'clock sharp.'

'Were there no other patients here?'

'Yes but Miss Woodruff showed me straight in.'

'Then you are out of turn and have kept a lot of other people waiting. Will you kindly go now and do as I've told you.' I walked to the door and held it open for her. She got up and went out without a word.

My annoyance was not so much at her as at Hannah

Woodruff. Mrs Bold was an easily understood soul who was afraid of cancer. She was probably scarcely aware that other people existed. Hannah Woodruff had once more given a number of patients justifiable reason for resentment.

At about quarter-past five a quiet gentle little man named Albert Strawman came in to see me. He lived in a neighbouring village and made his living as a smallholder who sold his produce to the local shops. He had acute synovitis of the knee. I put on a crepe bandage and told him he would have to rest a few days.

'Not gunner be easy to do thart zir,' he said. 'Oi gotter walk 'ome ver a ztart.'

I looked at my watch. There was still an evening bus to his village but he had missed it. 'Couldn't you have come earlier so as to catch the bus back?' I asked him.

'Oi did zir. Oi were yere at 'alf-past three.'

'Then why didn't you come in earlier?'

''Twere Miss Woodruff. She kep' tellin' other volks to come in.'

'Didn't you tell her it was your turn?'

'Didn't loike to really zir. Oi supposed they was more urgent cases loike.'

I became suddenly angry. This little man had been forced to wait long after his turn and now would have to walk home with a knee full of fluid. My temper snapped and I went out to the dispensary. I had never reproached Miss Woodruff in front of patients before but I was too angry now to consider this. 'Mr Strawman has been waiting since half-past three,' I said, 'and it's now twenty-past five. Why did you send all those other people in to see me out of turn?'

She looked surly and turned her back to me. 'And Mrs Bold arrived at four o'clock and you sent her in straight-away. Mr Strawman should have been seen an hour and a half ago and now he's missed his bus home. He's either got to walk home with a knee full of fluid or I shall have to drive him home when I've finished. And heaven knows when that will be. Very well, we'll talk about it in the morning.'

She knew she had gone too far this time and had the grace to murmur 'sorry'. I told her to send a message to the post office near Strawman's home and tell his wife he would be late, and then went on with my surgery. I finished at about eight o'clock and took Strawman home.

At last my mind was made up. Hannah Woodruff would have to go. I was sorry for her because the surgery had been her life, but I gave her notice the next day. Fortunately she found work with the opposition firm very quickly and vowed she would never set foot in our surgery again. She didn't.

In April 1941 I found Annabel Jamieson who made my life in the surgery a pleasure compared with what it had been for the previous twelve years. I was able to claim from her for many years all the help that a good secretary can give and my burden was enormously eased.

Two events of the remainder of 1941 stand out in the memory — the first of minor importance but interesting at the time, the second of major importance.

The first was the visit that summer from Professor Joad — famous on radio brains trusts for prefacing every answer with the words 'it all depends what you mean by —'. He came to Melbrook to lecture and we put him up. While we talked that evening Weston-super-mare was bombed and the hall where he was to have lectured the next evening was destroyed. He asked whether we could put him up for another night and of course we agreed. During the afternoon I took a few hours off and we went to Wells for a swim in the baths. No one of course recognised him, because in the days before television his medium had always been radio. His voice on the other hand and particularly his laugh were familiar to most people.

At one time he was floating on his back in the middle of the baths and the spectacle was quite funny. His somewhat generous abdomen emerged as a section of a sphere just out of the pool and from the region of his goatee beard three feet away there spurted from time to time small jets of chlorinated water. I made some remark which produced the typical Joad laugh, high-pitched and full of fun.

The effect was electric. Everyone in and around the baths knew at once who he was and they became suddenly silent. Some stared and some laughed before politeness took over again.

He retired to his bedroom after the swim to do some writing. I think the book he was working on at the time was his *God and Evil* but what I am quite sure of is that he used an old-fashioned pen which had to be dipped in the ink after every few words. His habit was to dip the pen in the ink and then flick off the excess on to the floor. Unfortunately we had rather a good carpet in that bedroom where he sat at a table under the window. The marks of the ink remained on it for some twenty years until it eventually wore out.

That evening we asked Edward Tyndall, vicar of a neighbouring parish and a good friend of mine, to join in our talk which I remember very well. We discussed evolution, life after death, the problem of pain to the Christian and the significance of conscience. Edward and I did our best to counter the arguments of Joad who was an atheist at that time. What interests me is that Joad in his book *Recovery of Belief* written some years later makes precise use of our arguments.

That night when Jessica and I went to bed she asked me what we had been talking about. 'Oh religion, God, evil, conscience, that sort of thing,' I said. 'He's an atheist of course.'

She lay back in her bath while I sat nearby. It was a regular time for talk about the day. 'What a waste of time arguing about it when it's all so obvious,' she said. 'We're ducks in a duckpond and can't see beyond the edge of the pond. That doesn't mean there's nothing else.'

I always envied her her wonderful faith in God, in prayer and in the power of loving kindness. It seemed that I worked very hard to find my way while all the time she was walking ahead with a lantern raised high. Why did I so often ask myself whether she really knew the way?

The major event of that year was the birth in September of our fourth baby. I attended the birth myself because there was no one else available that I would trust. This of course was not good practice but in wartime it seemed reasonable. Fortunately everything went well and that afternoon we were rewarded by the arrival of our daughter Beth.

Our family now seemed complete. We had always wanted and planned to have four children but we should have no more. Jessica enjoyed telling the story later of a plan suggested by the younger two children while I was overseas during the latter part of the war. They approached her solemnly one day and said, 'We think you ought to have another baby while Daddy is away. You could have a boy and it would be such a lovely surprise for him when he comes home.'

In the autumn of 1940 I had had the good fortune to find an elderly Portuguese Indian doctor to help in the practice. The work became lighter but in the spring of 1941 I was made medical officer of health for the district and some administration and committee work was added to the rest. All the same, during the winter of 1941/42 our routine became almost normal with the two of us working full time and Annabel Jamieson playing a big part in soothing our ways. Life was too good and too easy. Many of our great cities were being destroyed while we were as safe and comfortable as we were in peacetime. The worst of the war was clearly ahead of us and I felt that someone much older than I could do the work in Melbrook.

The problem was how to get someone to replace me. While we talked endlessly over the problem we heard that Tom Wyburn had been invalided home from Egypt with some skin trouble. The ideal solution to our problem would be to change places, but this seemed too simple and sensible a plan for the war machine to accomplish. Wyburn and I agreed that if I applied for enlistment to the R.A.M.C. and he applied simultaneously for release to run the practice it was just possible that some committee would be sane enough to do the right thing.

By some miracle this was how it worked out. I was in medical category A and Wyburn was C and the authorities made the brilliant decision that a unit of personnel in category A was more acceptable than a unit in category C.

So in May 1942 I joined the army.

4

The change from wartime general practice to life in the army was like going on holiday. But the holiday consisted of a planned sea and coach tour in which you had relinquished all control of your movements. We spent a few weeks in Church Crookham where several earnest sergeants did their utmost to discipline us but had to admit defeat.

This was not their fault. We were a group of middle-aged general practitioners who were enjoying freedom from responsibility for the first time for years. When you are suddenly freed from responsibility you become cheerful and relaxed, and this is not the best frame of mind for inducing you to make any serious effort to touch your toes many times over at six o'clock in the morning.

This stage of army life was marred only by our anti-typhoid injections. After these we had to walk out with temperatures of 103 or so and salute the 'other ranks' every few seconds with stiff painful right arms. It was one of the strange ways of the army that whereas other ranks had forty-eight hours off duty after their TAB inoculations, officers were expected to be made of such tough material that they could carry on regardless of swimming heads and paralysed right arms. I suppose the authorities planned this small discomfort to remind us that we were not really on holiday.

Several of us were posted to Peebles in Scotland where the best hotel — The Hydro — had been reserved for us for several months. A twelve hundred bedded hospital was being assembled there and we welcomed newcomers to the staff every few days. We walked and talked and got to

40

know each other and in August we shot grouse on the moors. I found the grouse very small and fast at first but they seemed to slow down after a week or so. I must admit I never really enjoyed shooting these lovely birds but as I seemed to be able to shoot fairly straight I went along with the others.

The Colonel was newly promoted and his rank sat none too easily on him. He was forced accordingly to remind us at fairly frequent intervals that he was in fact the commanding officer. His head was a little too small, his eyes a little too close together, and I had a little difficulty in hiding my dislike for him.

The mess was formal. There was no relaxation into the familiarity of Christian names and every officer was expected to address his seniors in rank at all times as 'sir'. The atmosphere made us wary of breaching the strange conventions of army life. Even after a drink or two members of the mess would move away in twos or threes for easier talk.

One evening the Colonel asked a group of us over a drink at the bar, 'Is there anyone here who can give anaesthetics?'

No one spoke and he went on, 'The staff anaesthetist won't be here for a month and we need someone to fill the gap. There won't be much to do but now we are equipped we shall have to do any surgery that turns up in this part of Scotland.'

Still no one spoke and I began to feel sorry for the poor chap, so I said tentatively that I had given anaesthetics from time to time in our cottage hospital at home and was quite prepared to help for a few weeks if necessary.

Before I knew where I was I had become the temporary unpaid hospital anaesthetist.

That evening I spoke to one of the surgeons. 'I'm no expert,' I said. 'I've simply given anaesthetics as part of my "jack-of-all-trades" experience.'

'You'll be alright,' replied the Major. 'If you stick to it you might get graded as an anaesthetist and that means promotion in time.'

'But I don't want to be an anaesthetist,' I said. 'I merely

offered to fill the gap until the proper chap arrives.'

'Ah. Then a bit of advice for you. Never volunteer for anything. It doesn't pay.'

During the next month I learnt the truth of his dictum.

I was introduced first of all to a huge Boyle's anaesthetic machine which looked the approximate size of my consulting-room in the surgery at home. I then learnt that every case had to be intubated — anaesthetised through a tube into the trachea itself. So I had to teach myself to introduce a tracheal tube which caused a good deal of delay at the beginning of each operation. Once this was done the ether could be given without difficulty in a stream of gas and oxygen direct into the trachea itself.

We had one or two operating sessions a week and the patients were all sturdy young men who took a good deal of knocking out but who were fairly tough material. After a week or two my main anxiety was that I might be trapped into becoming an anaesthetist for the duration of the war.

I made up my mind to see the Colonel about it and in due course I was shown into his room — some thirty feet square with a glorious view of the hills. I saluted smartly and stood at attention in front of his desk.

'I've come to see you about doing anaesthetics sir,' I said. 'I volunteered to fill a gap until the anaesthetist arrived but I don't want to go on indefinitely. Now that Major Curtis has arrived may I be transferred to the medical division?'

'Why don't you want to do anaesthetics? Curtis can't go on doing them all when we are in a theatre of war. He will need help.'

'I'm not an expert and frankly they bore me.' This was the truth but quite the wrong approach.

He looked at me with distaste. 'I understand you are *reasonably* competent at them.' He stressed the word reasonably. 'Do you really think that because you are *bored*' (another emphasis) 'by doing your duty, I should try to find something better suited to your taste?'

'I'm only asking to do what I'm best qualified to do, sir. I'm not a very good anaesthetist and I think I could be more use in the medical division.'

42

'If I have any complaints about your work I shall send for you. Alright, you may go.'

I knew it was no good arguing so I saluted and left. It looked as though I was booked for anaesthetics and the longer I carried on with that particular job the more likely I was to be kept at it. Once we set up hospital in a theatre of war I should have no hope of a change.

I didn't like the Colonel. It seemed equally clear that he didn't like me. I thought him the sort of man who might have been a hard insensitive schoolmaster with a tendency to make great favourites of some of the smaller boys. I soon discovered how I had blotted my copybook. I had told him I didn't play bridge and he had discovered that I did. I had been warned that if I admitted liking the game I should be committed to spending many hours at it whenever he commanded my presence.

By this time the medical division was fully assembled and I became keener than ever to join it. The O.C. Medical Division was Lt.Colonel Richardson and the medical specialist was Major Harman — both physicians on the staff of St Thomas' Hospital and men of the highest repute. What was more, they were the sort of men I wanted to work with. John Richardson had a combination of strength and sensitivity that I liked at once and John Harman was a good talker, witty and a stimulating companion. I soon recognised enough of their quality to become obsessed with the idea of joining them. I felt an outcast in the somewhat drab surgical division where the personalities were not so interesting.

One day I got hold of John Richardson, told him my problem and asked if he could help. He was obviously a man who suffered fools badly and was at first somewhat intimidating. I had to screw up my courage to ask a favour of him. To my great relief he was kindness itself and let me ramble on about my dislike of anaesthetics and my interest in medicine. To my surprise he already knew my past history — jobs at Guy's and experience in practice. He looked profoundly thoughtful and very serious for a moment while I waited for his reply.

Then he said, 'You'd better make a mess of a few anaesthetics, hadn't you?'

Not knowing him I thought he was being serious and looked at him in puzzled surprise. Then the hard glint in his eye suddenly changed and he burst out laughing. It was like the sun coming out on a stormy day. 'Don't take me too seriously,' he said. 'I'll have a word with the O.C. Surgical Div. and see if anything can be arranged.'

By September I had been rescued from anaesthetics and was a general duty officer in the medical division, with the prospect of the care of fifty out of the six hundred beds under the supervision of my two heroes.

Early in October we had embarkation leave, and as embarkation became imminent most of us had our wives to stay in the district and shared their lodgings. I had Jessica all to myself for ten days and we lived in our own heaven. We stayed with a charming lady named Mrs Anderson who was determined to fill our lives with as much good food and as much pleasure as possible. Her house was full of clocks, all registering different times, and when we asked which one was right she told us solemnly that they all were. Perhaps this added to our sense of the timelessness of those few days — our last together for two and a half years. Towards the end of the month I saw a tearful Jessica off at Peebles station and fell into the deepest pit of wretchedness I can ever remember.

A few days later we embarked on the P. and O. ship *Strathalan* at Greenock and on an early November evening we moved in an impressive line of twenty-three great ships down the Clyde. I shared a tiny cabin with two other officers of my rank — Rankin and Devereux — good companions of many months. We had two bunks and took turns to sleep on the floor until I decided I actually preferred the floor and kept to it. The only disadvantage was the descent of Rankin's large foot on my head every morning as he emerged from his bunk.

The ship had 'gone dry' only a month before and there were no alcoholic drinks available. Mess parties on the last night of previous voyages had done so much damage that we had to suffer for the sins of our predecessors.

The convoy headed west into the Atlantic but by that time we knew where we were going. We were part of the

First Army due to land in North Africa. The sea looked angry and dark and most of us were seasick during one bout of rough weather. We were guarded by four corvettes and a destroyer which seemed remarkably thin protection for such a large convoy, but compared with convoy duty on the Murmansk runs to Russia our guardians were on something of a pleasure trip. They certainly gave us confidence as the voyage proceeded. Every now and then a corvette would dart through the convoy, stop suddenly and appear to listen for a moment, then dash off in another direction and finally fire off depth charges which presumably chased away marauding submarines. They resembled lively terriers excited by the prospect of a rat somewhere nearby.

On the fourth day out I read in the day's orders that I was to 'F.F.I.' the troops on one section of one of the decks. I discovered there were something like seven hundred of them. As I set about the task I found that the 'other ranks' were far less comfortably billeted than we were. They slept tightly packed in hammocks or on the floor. The air was foul with the smell of vomit and sweat. I merely had to work there for a few hours; they had to sleep there.

'F.F.I.' meaning freedom from infestation, entails a brief examination of each man which experienced army medical officers get through in about ten seconds. It is a humiliating affair for the men. They appear before you stark naked with their arms held up and you examine the skin of the arms, legs, and back and front of the body. You run your hands over the skin to feel any irregularities which might be produced by scabies and look for bite marks from lice or fleas. I was probably too conscientious and spent many hours over my seven hundred, finally signing papers with lists of names on them which were presented to me by various N.C.O.s. It wasn't exactly a thrilling piece of war work. In fact it was about the most menial task in the army medical world.

We proceeded west, then south and then east again, approaching Gibraltar after about a week. On the seventh evening a message came through that 'large numbers of

45

enemy submarines are assembling near the Straits of Gibraltar. A rough time must be prepared for.' The message was, I remember, greeted by raucous laughter, for by that time our confidence in our escort was absolute. Nothing could happen to us, to others perhaps, but not to us. As it happened we went through the Straits and on into Algiers harbour quite unharmed, but that was where the trouble began in the shape of air bombardment.

There was only one undamaged landing dock, so we could only unload one ship at a time while the Germans used us for target practice. Most of the attacks came by night and on the second night, while we were still awaiting our turn to disembark, John Harman and I were detailed to prepare a ward for casualties deep in the bowels of the ship below the water line. In air attack as opposed to torpedo attack this was the safest place. We did what we could by way of preparations, which wasn't much, and then settled down to wait. Nothing happened and as John Harman was wide awake I decided to go to sleep — something I am fairly good at. Between two and three in the morning the Colonel came to see us and I awoke to see him bending over me. Harman stood behind him, suppressing his laughter, but my first thought was that the C.O. looked as though he intended to have me shot for sleeping on duty.

I don't think my situation was serious but I shall never know, because at that moment the constant noise of bombs suddenly exploded into something very close to the ship which shuddered violently. The Colonel left us briskly to find out what had happened and presently we were told to stay where we were. No casualties appeared, but in the morning we saw that the ship next to us had been cut in half, exposing much of its inside, but still afloat. The *Strathalan* was untouched. Her turn was still to come.

Our disembarkation took a long time and we seemed to litter a huge area with packages and equipment and thousands of khaki-clad figures moving like ants in all directions. It was nightfall by the time we were ready to start on our journey to Ben Aknoun where we were to set up hospital, so we were marched out of Algiers and told to 'make ourselves comfortable' in a field to the west of the city.

It was soon pitch dark and beginning to rain. It was also very cold. We ate our rations, consisting of some biscuits and a packet of delicious solid oatmeal which was sweet and well salted, creating the illusion for a time of a full stomach. We wrapped ourselves in our ground sheets but before long the rain was coming down in torrents.

Some of the young 'other ranks' put their helmets over their faces and appeared to go into a sound sleep. I admired and envied them but had no hope of sleep myself, and realised that I was not so tough as I had thought. There is a vast difference between the toughness of twenty and that of thirty-six. About midnight I was so cold that I began to wander round. There was a building at the end of the field and I looked into it. There was room for twenty or more bodies to lie down there and it seemed a pity not to make the most of it. Just as I was settling down the Colonel came out from somewhere and asked me what I was doing. The thought struck me that this man was either engaging in a personal vendetta against me, or was having me spied on so as to be made aware of the slightest irregularity in my behaviour.

I told him it seemed silly to lie out in the rain when there was shelter available but this somehow made him very angry.

'Is there any reason why junior officers should be treated with special favour? We can't get the whole unit in here so you must share the same conditions as the men. Go along.'

What he said sounds quite reasonable as I write it, but wet through and half-frozen I took a different view of his orders. I spent the rest of the night trying to keep some sort of circulation in existence in the hope that the morning would see me still alive.

We took a roundabout route of what was said to be fifteen miles to Ben Aknoun, and having no personnel transport we carried our packs on our backs. I remember going up a long hill, several hundred miles long, which climbed along the side of a valley appropriately named the valley of the 'Femmes Sauvages'. We reached the disused school at nightfall. This was to be the basis of our hospital. The floor was dry and our boots made fair pillows. Compared with the previous night it was luxury.

We awoke next morning to something like fairyland. The sun shone and orange trees were loaded with fruit, not quite ripe but a treat nevertheless because we hadn't seen an orange for over two years. Hospital beds were prepared in the buildings and staff were accommodated in tents in the grounds. We were at last in action in a theatre of war.

One evening before Christmas one of the younger general duty officers put his head into the tent I shared with Devereux. He looked excited. 'Have you heard the news?'

'No. The war ended or something?'

'Better than that. Our nurses are expected here next week.'

Devereux was a serious man of strict virtue. 'So what?' he said.

'Won't you enjoy seeing a nice shape or two,' he made sweeping movements of his hands to indicate curves, 'instead of nothing but bloody males everywhere?'

'You keep your mind on your work, young fellow,' said Devereux, 'and leave the girls alone.'

Personally I welcomed the news. I always enjoy feminine company and the prospect of some sociability was cheering.

The next news we had of our nurses was that they had travelled out on the *Strathalan* which had been sunk a hundred miles off Algiers. All the nurses except two were picked up and arrived two days later. Their plight was sad to see. They had lost all their belongings and had been issued with ill-fitting men's battle dresses. After being in the sea there was not a tidy head of hair among them but they were remarkably cheerful. The only complaint I heard was that being made seasick by the waves while you were struggling to keep afloat was 'rather unpleasant'.

Our first cases on the medical side — some of the saddest I had ever seen — were thirty young men whose nerves had been shattered by the bombing at Bone. They were a pathetic sight. They grimaced, stammered, their limbs jerked and it seemed that their bodies were completely out of control. Their flat masklike faces seemed to indicate minds that had abdicated all pretence to life or contact with reality. At Bone they had been bombed continually for several days and had run out of ammunition for anti-aircraft defence. I hadn't realised the extent to which ac.ac. defences keep up the morale of those under attack. So long as you are hitting back you feel you have a chance to survive, but without any defence the nerves have to be made of steel to withstand attack for hour after hour and day after day.

·We gave them strong sedation but couldn't help them much. All were invalided back to the U.K. in due course.

We worked hard through the spring and summer, the beds being full of cases of malaria and dysentery. In February I heard the cuckoo. In March I was made 'malaria officer' which entailed walking over the countryside for some miles round Ben Aknoun and plotting the position of every smallest puddle of still water where mosquitoes might breed. I enjoyed these times alone as much as any in North Africa.

One evening I was sent for to see a new batch of cases that had arrived from the battle area to the east of us. Most of them on the medical side were routine cases of malaria or dysentery and were fairly quickly dealt with. Then I came to one with a Somerset accent.

'Which part of Somerset?' I asked him.

'Outside o' Wells.'

He was a stretcher case and before I examined him I talked to him for a few minutes. It was mainly for the pleasure of hearing him speak and I warmed to him with every rounded vowel sound. He was plainly glad to talk to someone from near his own home, but as soon as I asked about his trouble his face clouded with anxiety.

'Tis these legs o' mine', he said. 'Most 'en paralysed they do say.'

I looked at his notes and he was labelled 'poliomyelitis'. This was sad news. I discovered that his paralysis was still developing which meant that the outlook was serious.

As soon as I had gone over the rest of the intake I came back to him and he asked the pointed question, 'Do 'e reckon I be goin' to walk agen?' For a moment real fear showed in his face and I cursed the fate that this, of all our patients, should be a polio victim. His legs were severely paralysed and his right arm and shoulder muscles were affected too.

The diagnosis was not certain because we had had a few cases of acute infective polyneuritis — a condition I had never met before — so I examined him very carefully. There is no loss of sensation in poliomyelitis and I tested his skin sensitivity with the utmost care.

To my enormous relief there were clear signs that he was a case of infective polyneuritis. This would mean that he would probably recover completely. I knew I ought to be cautious until I had had another opinion, but within a few minutes I had told him I thought he was going to recover.

He looked at me as though he thought I was trying to buoy him up by deception. 'You mean I haven't got this infantile paralysis?'

'I'm pretty sure you haven't. And that means you will recover completely. I'll get one of the specialists to see you in the morning.'

'I can't 'ardly believe thart. Not that I'll get prarperly better. 'Tis too good to be true. What do 'e reckon 'tis then?' He held up his weak right arm.

As we talked I found the combination of hope and anxiety in his expression really moving. There was no sign of weakness in his respiratory muscles, and beyond ordering careful observation of these there was nothing more to be done that night. I prayed to heaven that I was right and hadn't raised false hopes.

Next day the diagnosis was confirmed by the O.C. Medical Division and I breathed a sigh of relief. Over the next few weeks there was steady improvement and I had the pleasure of demonstrating his case to a combined round of physicians. For some reason I was inordinately proud, not only of my diagnosis, but of the natural cure that followed. It was touch and go whether he was sent back to the U.K. or to convalescence and then duty. I did my best to have him put on the U.K. list and two months later he left us for England.

I gave him messages for Jessica which he faithfully delivered by telephone as soon as he got back to Somerset on leave. In his pleasure at being home he flattered my reputation with complete lack of justification but enormous good will, and Jessica of course was delighted.

When we had any time off that summer we went sailing — Devereux, Rankin and I. Devereux was a skilled sailor and we hired a good sized boat. One perfect summer evening the *King George the Fifth* was in dock in Algiers Harbour as we sailed in. From the radio of the great battleship the notes of Beethoven's Moonlight Sonata floated across the still water. It was hard to imagine that the ship could ever fire her guns in anger.

Two of us were invited to dine in the mess of one of the destroyers one evening and I remember crossing a sort of bridge of small ships lying side by side, with narrow planks joining each deck to the next. We had no trouble on our outward journey but I had my doubts about the homeward trip after several alcoholic hours with the Royal Navy. Strangely enough we skipped over those planks on the way back with no trouble at all, blissfully unaware of the thirty-foot drop into black sea that would receive you if you put a foot off the twelve-inch plank. Sweet are the uses of rum and milk, passed round in a communal cup with a towel to wipe away the inevitable sweat that followed each draught.

John Richardson was appointed physician in charge of the Royal party when King George the Sixth came out to North Africa. Afterwards he was awarded the M.V.O. — the first of the many honours which the years were to bring him and which took him finally to the House of Lords.

He told us of the King's departure. A message was sent to London stating the time he would leave Algiers. Later, when the intelligence service received the information that — as had been intended — this message had been picked up by the Germans, his time of departure was changed by several hours. He arrived safely in London in due course.

The sad epilogue to the story was that a British plane travelling between Portugal and London at the time the Germans had expected the king to be in the air was intercepted and brought down. It was carrying the actor Leslie Howard.

Before the end of the summer John Richardson sent for me and told me my grading had come through. He had told me he had recommended it some time before. This was tremendous news as it gave me consultant status and much more responsibility. I could now write after the signature on my reports, 'Capt. Graded Physician'. The disadvantage was that I should be posted to another hospital where I could take on the job and responsibility of medical specialist. I was in fact soon posted to a six hundred bedded hospital in Phillipville. Before I left, the Colonel sent for me.

'So you were right after all, Lane. You are more use in the medical division. Congratulations and good luck.' He shook hands with me and I thought perhaps he wasn't such a bad chap after all.

I didn't see him again. He was killed by a land mine which blew up his jeep some months later.

My good luck held because my new O.C. Medical Division was none other than Lt. Colonel Platt, well-known physician, later Brigadier Platt, later President of the Royal College of Physicians, and later still Lord Platt. We worked in harmony and he continued my medical education for eighteen months. Away from the wards we played chess a good deal and I heard at first hand most of the famous Platt stories. These I will not repeat because they belong very much to him and many were published some time before his death in his book *Private and Controversial*.

One of his valuable pieces of advice was, 'Always listen carefully to the patient's opinion of his illness. He is often right.' I learnt this and much more from this wise man.

It was quite remarkable that the first two of my medical chiefs in the army should have reached in later years the pinnacle of medical achievement. Both John Richardson and Robert Platt became distinguished presidents of the College.

While I was with this hospital my majority came through and I was at last able to have crowns put on the shoulders of my battle dress. By this time I was in charge of a good section of the medical division and was doing regular out-patient sessions to deal with men sent in from other units. Life was full and interesting.

Jessica wrote to me nearly every day throughout my army service. Her letters arrived in batches and had to wait till I could be alone somewhere to absorb them thoroughly. The doings of the children were recorded fully but none of the problems. Messages between the lines that only I could read kept my morale as high as possible. It was impossible to keep all her letters and by destroying them I lost a source of information about home life that was irreplaceable. My letters home half-filled a huge chest. We burned them one day in 1960 and have regretted their destruction ever since.

After the Salerno landings I had one of my periodic bouts of conscience. Life was too easy. If I had to be away from home — the only real hardship — why was I not doing more? I volunteered to go to Salerno where they were hard pressed and in need of anaesthetists, but when I talked this over with Robert Platt he refused to pass my offer on to the authorities. It was some time before my mind was easy but at least I could tell myself that I had tried. Perhaps my epitaph should be 'He meant well but was not very determined'.

The problem of conscience was complicated by a conflict of loyalties. I wasn't sure whether I ought to rush into uncalled-for dangers while I had a wife and four children at home. I certainly wasn't brave but I honestly wanted to take some share of the risks that so many were being forced to run. The main advantage of service life was that you had no real need of a conscience, you just did as you were told.

In February 1944 we were moved to Naples, arriving to see Vesuvius snow-covered but the Bay as lovely as ever. It was the height of the typhus epidemic there and my first memory of Naples is of the daily elaborate funerals. The people were poverty-stricken but nothing would prevent them from spending all they had on the six plumed white horses that took them to their graves. Preventive measures

53

consisted of blowing powder under the clothing of each individual Italian to kill the lice that were carrying the disease. The whole population went about with marks of white powder on necks, skirts and trousers. In three weeks the epidemic died out.

Our own casualties were mainly from the ferocious battle of Monte Cassino some miles to our north, but on the medical side we had only routine cases to deal with. Rome fell on D-day and after this Italian resistance crumbled, Mussolini was assassinated and the end drew nearer.

It was here that 'Lili Marlene' caught up with us, conveyed I suppose by the Eighth Army veterans who had taken it from the German Desert Army. The song's sadness increased one's homesickness but there was hope in the air now. Of course there were some depressing souls who insisted that we should be posted to the Far East direct from the Mediterranean and should be there for at least ten years. As one who had been saying ever since I entered the army that home leave was only six months away, my own forecast was by then discredited.

I had leave in September 1944 and hitch-hiked to Assissi where I visited the Hermitage. I was shown the exact hole in the ground where the devil disappeared when St Francis banished him, and when I admired the lovely little wild cyclamen flowers under the trees one of the monks dug up a dozen of the corms for me to take away. I posted them home and they still bloom in our garden.

In March 1945 we began our journey to north-west Europe by way of Marseilles and then by truck to Ghent. Most of France was liberated and the atmosphere was changing every day. People were in festive mood everywhere and we were counting the weeks till we should be given home leave.

This came fittingly on V.E. day when I crossed the Channel in calm and lovely weather and then made my way home for seven days.

Jessica met me at Bath Station and we drove home to Melbrook. The familiar hills, the lovely countryside, the roads laced on each side with cow parsley were as enchanting as ever. Nothing had changed. I remembered complaining in the mess one evening, during the darkest days in North Africa, that by the time we got home my wife would be getting on for forty. I needn't have worried. She hadn't changed.

At home there was a rapturous welcome from the four girls — all home from school for the occasion. Then I remember Beth, who was four, saying plaintively to her mother, 'Is he *their* daddy too?' She had only known me as a head and shoulders photograph in uniform to which she had said goodnight regularly as long as she could remember, and of course she regarded me as her own personal property.

The last stage of my overseas war service was in Norway. I went with the thirtieth General Hospital to Tromso in the Arctic Circle where we had the grisly task of rescuing Russian prisoners of war who had been starved by the Germans.

Most of these had died or returned to Russia. We had to attempt to resuscitate those who were too ill to travel. They were a pitiful sight, akin to the victims of Belsen and Auschwitz. They had been reduced to the desperation of eating the flesh of their own dead and one of our duties was to collect the evidence of their cannibalism to present to the War Crimes Tribunal.

After the war against the Japanese ended in August I worked in Shenley in north London, where I saw all the men from the Far East — mostly ex-prisoners of the Japanese — who were suffering from tuberculosis. This aftermath of the grimmer aspects of the war was another painful reminder of the sufferings of others. It was a long time before I could forgive the Japanese for their atrocities. I did however learn a good deal about the treatment of tuberculosis that was available at that time — an experience that was to serve me in good stead at home.

On a May morning in 1946 — just four years after I had left — I arrived at Bath Station and was home for good.

5

Coming home at the end of my war service I was not met by the town band like my predecessor, Dr Ballard. The story was told that the band met him at Melbrook Station and led him in triumph through the High Street to his home. My welcome was quieter. An old friend and patient brought Jessica to meet me, and the tear in his eye as he made a fair attempt to amputate my right hand fitted my mood better than sounding brass.

It was nearly seven years since in August 1939 the family had set out on our last holiday together and been called back twenty-four hours later. Now at last we had plenty of time. The years seemed to stretch ahead of us in endless progression as we began to fill the hundreds of gaps in our communication caused by separation and censorship.

After a few days at home I went back to work. Tom Wyburn had been hard pressed these four years and needed relief without delay. I was very fit and ready to take on the world if necessary

There was a splendid atmosphere about that postwar period. In spite of strict rationing and the absence of anything remotely resembling luxury, there was a general cheerfulness. We were still united as one people and in spite of all the dismal prognostications we had proved ourselves once more a nation to be reckoned with. The Battle of Britain was still fresh in the memory and every man, woman and child had played a part in the defeat of Hitler's Germany. Even in 1947, on our first holiday abroad, we were welcomed and feted because we were British.

One of my first patients that May was a young woman I

will call Dinah Barrett. I had known and treated her since she was a small girl with long pigtails that flapped rhythmically as she trotted on her pony. In the years of my absence she had grown into an attractive young woman of twenty-two. Her boyfriend had just been demobbed from a parachute regiment and they were to be married shortly. Unlike many other couples they had postponed their marriage until they could settle down properly in their own home.

As I have said before, I am something of a romantic and the memory of these two stays with me. The combination of a fine young man with a splendid war record and a fresh, attractive girl was irresistibly appealing.

I saw them both one evening at the Barretts' house when I was called to see a younger sister who had injured her leg. We were less inclined in those days to use the hospital for every minor injury and I did my stitching in the house. Then I met Stephen for the first time and liked him. Dinah was a delightful girl, full of fun. There was no outward show of sentiment yet one felt the certainty of strong feelings between the two of them.

The marriage date was fixed for a couple of weeks ahead and the whole town was involved. It was to be the wedding of the year, a full choir in the church, a full peal of bells and a large reception at the Barretts' house. They were expecting two hundred guests which was a large number for a country wedding. Dinah was a registered nurse but had been at home for several months and active in the town. She had made a lot of friends and had invited all of them, from one end of the social scale to the other. Looking back to that evening when I stitched the sister's leg I remember two things about Dinah — her vitality and her clear, almost transparent complexion. She was a very efficient assistant too. My instruments were sterilised and cooled as if by magic and laid out on a sterile towel she had borrowed from the cottage hospital. Then without any effort on my part the patient was placed so as to allow perfect light on the cut, and easy access without twisting or breaking your back to do the job. Small things perhaps but for minor surgery in a house, quite important.

'You could probably do this every bit as well yourself, Dinah,' I said.

'For her?' She laughed. 'She wouldn't let me touch her. She's always telling me I'm a nurse and not a doctor.'

'Women often stitch better than men,' I replied.

'That's nonsense. Men are marvellous needleworkers when they can be bothered. Give me a man every time.'

The patient interrupted us. 'I'm dreading this. I wish you would get on with it.'

I promised not to hurt and took great care in putting local anaesthetic under the skin edge. 'Your sister is a very tactful girl,' I told her. 'She is putting me on my mettle.' And I determined to be especially careful to make a good job of the repair of the jagged four-inch cut. As soon as I had finished, Dinah had a neat dressing in place in no time and I was asked to stay for a glass of champagne. It was somebody's birthday — Stephen's I think. He would be twenty-eight or twenty-nine.

There were several strangers there and while I drank I talked to Stephen. I always felt that serving in the R.A.M.C. I was not a real soldier, but we exchanged wartime experiences for a time and then he led me out on to the lawn.

'I want to ask you about Dinah,' he said. 'I'm not sure she is well. I've been here several days now and although she pretends to be full of life she gets suddenly tired and irritable. It's not like her. Last year I was here on leave and she would stay up late at night and still be ready for anything next day.'

'Pre-wedding nerves,' I suggested.

'I'm not sure.'

'If you're worried can you get her to come and see me?'

'She went to see your deputy before you came home and he said she was alright but I'd be glad if you would check her up.'

'Of course I will. I'll examine her here at the house if she likes.'

'She has lost some weight too.'

'Girls always lose weight before they are married,' I reassured him. 'She's probably feeling the normal strain.

58

Anyway you'll make sure she sees me? I can't do much unless she makes a move herself.'

'I'll make sure of that.'

He was such a solid character that I took his anxiety seriously. I looked up her notes and it was evident that the assistant — who had left when I came home — had made a careful examination and found nothing wrong. On the other hand Dinah must have made that appointment herself without any prodding from Stephen, and this must mean something.

She came to see me at the surgery the next day. She admitted to feeling tired at times but nothing else. I examined her carefully but found nothing wrong.

I had spent the last few months of my army service at Shenley where I saw all the chest cases returning from the Far East. Many were ex-prisoners of war of the Japanese and some were very ill. A large number had tuberculosis and we treated these with the few surgical procedures available at the time — artificial pneumothorax, division of adhesions as well as an occasional thoracoplasty. My mind ran naturally on the lines of tuberculosis and I told Dinah we would get an Xray of her chest as a routine precaution.

As she dressed, she asked me if I could hear anything, which suggested that her thoughts had been similar to mine.

'Not a thing,' I said. 'We'll have a chest Xray and a blood test and if they are both normal I won't trouble you any more. A good holiday with Stephen should put you right.'

The Xray showed what was almost certainly active tuberculosis in one lung.

I was shocked. All the appalling implications came crowding on me — these vile fuzzy shadows, the poison and the germs were already spreading through the body, the slow inexorable spread that would eventually kill her.

It is one thing to find tuberculosis in a stranger but quite another to find it in someone you know and like. What now? And what about the wedding?

The blood test showed evidence of active infection of

some sort and the sputum test would probably give proof of active tuberculosis. While I waited for this I should at least have time to think. But the more I thought the worse things seemed. Should they marry as planned or must I advise them to cancel the wedding to the distress of the family — and the whole town for that matter. It was important to make an exact diagnosis but there was little doubt about this already. The sputum test would make it absolute. If that were positive Dinah would have to rest for some months in any case — probably a year — then a life of semi-invalidism was the best she could hope for.

The impact of his particular tragedy — the discovery of tuberculosis — was harsh and shattering in those days. Not long before, it was a death sentence worse than cancer. It was more agonising to watch and to suffer because it was so much more prolonged.

I suppose I was more distressed over this disease because as a child I had watched my mother die of it. Her 'consumption' was diagnosed when I was five and after a family conclave it was decided that I, the youngest, whose schooling would not be affected should go with her to Margate where the sea air would do her good. The next three years were bad ones for me and I hated every minute of them.

Only in recent years had some hope been offered by the surgical treatment of thoracoplasty. Dinah knew this all too well and when I had the positive sputum result I could put off a straight talk with her no longer.

I discussed everything with Stephen first. He must have been shattered by the news yet I felt he was in some way prepared for it. So often in general practice the giving of bad news is made easier because the patient has half-suspected the truth beforehand.

When I told Stephen that Dinah would have to rest for a year and might have to undergo major surgery he took the news with apparent calm and stoicism but in absolute silence. 'What are the ultimate chances?' he asked.

'The best hope is thoracoplasty — an operation to collapse the affected part of the lung so as to control the spread of the disease. It's being done more and more and with a good deal of success.'

60

'I don't want the wedding postponed,' he said. 'I must have responsibility for her whatever happens. We can be married and she can go straight to hospital the same day instead of on a honeymoon. Would she come to any harm by carrying on till then? It's only a fortnight. Alternatively they could just cancel the reception.'

One has to guard against becoming too emotionally involved with patients, but sometimes it is very difficult. When you are young, you are too full of your own affairs to be over much affected but as you get older you can easily live too close to your patients' pain. I hated this awful disease — the increasing fever, the body-shaking cough, the pain in the chest, the constant night sweats and the exhaustion, all punctuated by the piercing thrusts of sudden haemorrhage. To think that this lovely girl must face all this was enough to make you rave bitterly against the vileness of nature and the world in general.

I understoood Stephen's feelings very well. He loved Dinah and his love meant suffering which he was fully prepared for. He didn't say a word about his own disappointment. His physical need of her after years of war and danger would be intense but was put entirely in the background. He insisted on breaking the news to Dinah himself.

That evening, while I was wrapped in gloom, the most traumatic experience of my own childhood came forcibly back to me. I sat again in the classroom of my father's school. I was eight years old. We had a teacher named Miss Templeton whom I worshipped from a distance. She must have been about twenty-one or twenty-two and was very pretty. I remember her calling me out of class and taking me to another room. There she put her arms round me and kissed me, surrounding my world with a golden haze. Then she told me my father wanted to talk to me and was waiting for me outside. He took my hand and we walked together towards our house. I was still in a happy dream. Then when we reached a certain stile near the bottom of Bolt's Hill he said, 'Your dear mother has died now. She is not in any more pain.' It was a long time before the news sank in, but when we reached the house I knew something terrible had happened. For months afterwards I was in what I now recognise must have been a deep infantile depression. At least Dinah had no children.

I hoped Stephen would have his way over the wedding but I reckoned without Dinah. I had a long talk with her the next day when she had had time to get over the shock of the news. I stressed the good prospects of rest and surgery, telling her that in a year she might be able to start married life properly. Then I praised Stephen. 'He wants you to go ahead with the wedding and then go straight to hospital,' I said.

She shook her head. 'No, I won't do that.'

'You mean you won't go to hospital, but you must Dinah.'

'I'll go to hospital but I won't marry Stephen.'

There was a silence so fully charged that it seemed wrong to break it. What more could usefully be said? Her expression was not in any way resigned but it was utterly determined. Since Stephen had broken the news to her she had thought the whole problem through. She had made up her mind but couldn't put her reasons or her feelings into words.

'He wants to be responsible for you,' I said presently.

'He's not going to marry an invalid. If things go well — very well — he may wait for me. I don't know. I shan't expect him to.'

'I think you have underestimated him. If you won't marry him now he'll wait.'

Then she became practical. 'May I see the Xrays?'

'Of course.' I showed her the films. The area of shadow at the apex of one lung looked mild enough and I made no comment.

'It doesn't look too bad,' she remarked.

'It isn't too bad. A thoracoplasty would shut up that area and it would heal.'

Another silence as she gazed at the picture of her lungs. Presently we talked of practical plans. I told her whom I wanted her to see and that I hoped to get her into the King Edward the Seventh Hospital at Midhurst in Sussex.

'What a long way away,' she said.

'It's the best place. A marvellous hospital and a splendid staff.'

'I haven't seen what people look like after a thoracoplasty. Does it ruin the figure?'

'No. The shoulders are kept in position and the breasts are hardly affected. No one would know when you are dressed.'

'And when you are undressed?'

'Nothing that would worry Stephen.'

The atmosphere began to lighten between us. The early stages of tuberculosis have one curious effect on the patient. There is often a euphoria, an illogical optimism against the odds. Perhaps this came to our rescue.

'I feel better for talking about it,' Dinah told me, and a deep slow breath was the outward sign of a degree of relaxation.

'You are quite decided about postponing the wedding? Stephen is very keen on your being married now and there is a lot to be said for it. You may feel you want him to be free, but he's not going to feel free anyway. His feelings for you won't change and if you are to be married later, why not now if he wants it? Besides, you could have a day or two together.'

'Don't tempt me. I've been thinking about it most of the night. If I thought it was hopeless I would know what to do, but I'm hoping I can offer him a more healthy wife in a year's time. There's hope of that, isn't there?'

'Of course there is.' I had to be optimistic but my doubts weighed heavily. 'What are your real reasons for putting it off?'

'He'd be giving me so much and I'd be giving him so little. What is the good of a wife in a sanatorium? I suppose it's pride but I can't help it.'

To have pressed any more would have been giving away my doubts about the outcome of her illness. 'Ask me to the wedding next summer then,' I said.

Before she left she asked one more question. 'Could I have given it to Stephen?'

'It's not at all likely. I'm having him Xrayed as a contact, as well as your sister and the rest of the family. I'm sure Stephen is alright.'

The wedding was cancelled. The shock waves of the news

died down in a week or so and I believe the wedding presents were kept in the hope that it was only a postponement. Time passed and Dinah's mother suffered, I think, as much as she did. The thoracoplasty was performed and she improved remarkably.

They were married eighteen months later with strict orders that there were to be no children. The disease was still latent.

Three years later came the glorious news that a combination of three antibiotics was curing tuberculosis. The impossible had happened. The one disease I had told myself would never be cured medically was brought under control. When I think of it, I am profoundly grateful that I have lived when I have. No one can appreciate the wonders of modern medicine who has not seen and lived through the horrors that existed without them.

Dinah had a long course of antibiotics and was eventually pronouncd cured. She had two babies both of whom are now healthy young adults.

Theirs is a good marriage — but then they are both good people. I gave up long ago believing that mankind consists of nothing but 'grey' individuals, neither good nor bad. Absolutes in human nature don't exist, but all the same there are some very good people and some very bad ones.

6

When Annabel Jamieson had replaced Hannah Woodruff as our secretary dispenser in 1941 the atmosphere of the surgery changed dramatically. Annabel, or Miss Jamieson as we called her for many years, liked both Tom Wyburn and me, kept us strictly in order and used a combination of tact and personality to keep all tension out of the place. When I say she kept us in order I mean this literally, though it would take a lot of space to explain exactly how. In general practice there are times when patients can be thoroughly irritating. The day after you have had a long and worrying night call, for instance, may be exactly the day that your most vocal patient has the first appointment and makes you half an hour late for the rest of the day; or the morning you have a painful attack of laryngitis may be the very day that all your deaf patients consult you one after another. At these times an understanding secretary, who is able to damp down all unreasonable reactions on your part, does a valuable job.

Perhaps as a direct reaction against the ways of her predecessor, Annabel always managed to keep the parish and club patients at the top of the priority list. When she handed us our visiting lists, for instance, these poorer folk would be at the top and the private patients at the bottom. She once justified this habit by saying 'look after the pence and the pounds will look after themselves' — appealing to a nice balance of morality and self-interest on our part.

Before penicillin came into general use, the sulphonamide drugs were our most cherished weapon. They were used against all manner of infections, sometimes with dramatic effect. These first of the wonder drugs were, of course, tried on every type of infection, many of which were completely resistant to them. I remember one enthusiast who tried them in a case of cancer.

Miss Jamieson asked me one day how much we were to charge for surgery attendance and medicine when sulphonamide tablets were prescribed.

'How much do they cost?' I asked.

'Sixteen and six a hundred. That's about tuppence each.' She waited patiently for me to understand.

'I see. So we charge four shillings for attendance and medicine, and when we give sulphonamide tablets we usually prescribe forty, which would cost us eighty pence, which is six and eightpence. So we lose two shillings and eightpence on each consultation. We shan't get very rich doing that.'

'You can't possibly go on like that, Doctor. It's outrageous.'

'But putting up the charge for attendance and medicine will cause a revolution. It's been the same since the beginning of time and probably longer.'

'Why don't you charge three shillings and sixpence for the consultation and let them pay for the medicine separately?'

'That would mean charging three and sixpence plus six and eightpence which is nine and twopence —'

'Ten and tuppence, Doctor.'

'Ten and tuppence. A lot of people won't be able to afford that. How often do we prescribe sulphonamide — say in a week?'

'Ten to fifteen times a week in the winter months.'

'And every time we do, we lose six and eightpence. That's about nine or ten pounds a week. I'll talk to Dr Wyburn about it.'

'Fifteen times six and eightpence would be five pounds,' Miss Jamieson corrected me.

A day or two later Wyburn and I discussed the matter. The loss of five pounds a week would be equivalent to a hundred a week in 1982, but even so I half-expected him to brush it on one side. He believed firmly that money looked after itself. There always seemed to the plenty rolling in to

66

keep us going. To my surprise he was shocked.

'I had no idea these sulphonamides were so expensive,' he said. 'We shall have to put up a notice explaining our dilemma. I don't like discussing money with patients but we can't go on like this.'

I told him of Miss Jamieson's suggestion that we should charge three and six for the consultation plus the cost of the medicine or tablets.

'Then what do we do when they have a simple bottle of medicine? How much does a bottle of mist. pot. brom. cost, for instance?'

'The ingredients would cost about sixpence and the bottle tuppence. The dispensing fee would be the biggest item — say one and sixpence — that would be two and tuppence altogether.'

'So if we suddenly charge three and six for the consultation plus, say, two and six for the medicine, this would mean putting up the charge for attendance and medicine from four shillings to six shillings. An increase of fifty percent. We can't possibly do that.'

'Suppose we charge three and six for attendance plus one and six for medicine, or six and eightpence when they have sulphonamide.'

'How complicated. No one would ever understand that. People always think they are paying the whole charge for the medicine and nothing for the consultation.'

'They've got to be educated,' I said firmly.

Wyburn concentrated hard for a moment. 'I think a round charge of five shillings for attendance and medicine. Then we should gain enough on the majority of attendances to pay for the loss when people had sulphonamides.'

'Then everyone would say we had put up our charges for nothing. It would be better to keep the charge at four shillings and make an extra charge of say six shillings when they have sulphonamides.'

The simplicity and round figures seemed to appeal to Wyburn. He went for a moment into one of his trance-like states but finally we agreed on this procedure.

The actual original of this discussion lasted for at least

three long sessions but the gist of the argument was as I have indicated. We felt instinctively that the decision was epoch-making and so it turned out. Similar decisions all over the country set our steps firmly and inevitably on the weary road to inflation.

It was only a few days before trouble broke out in the person of a man I will call Bob Toddy. The name suits him better than his own. Bob was a miniature version of Sam Weller with a Somerset accent. He was thin and wiry with a very shrewd eye for a bargain. He called himself a dealer, which meant that he sold anything from an old iron bedstead to a sack of manure. His wife had been prescribed sulphonamide tablets for an acute ear infection and had been asked to pay an extra six shillings. Bob demanded to see me and I talked to him in the waiting-room. I thought it would save time if as many people as possible heard the reasons for the charge, and the word would get round that we were not making an excess profit.

Bob rattled the tablets in their box. 'They'm pretty expensive, bain't they zir?'

'They are, Bob, but they cost us more than that.'

For a moment he was nonplussed. He was used to telling people that he was selling at cost price. He had used that sort of language to his customers scores of times. But to hear someone claim they were selling at less than cost price was clearly a lie. Much worse, it was a lie that anyone would notice. His face relaxed and he winked at me, then dropped his voice. 'No one can do business like that, Doctor, now can they? Not less than cost price. What do they really cost? I won't repeat it mind. Say two bob?'

I couldn't help laughing at him and repeated that they cost us exactly six shillings and eightpence.

He turned round in a complete circle which was a curious habit he had while 'doing business'. 'Oi understand zir. Oi *underztand*. Oi'm a business marn tew. Couldn't we zettle ver a bit less loike? Zay 'arf a crown?'

'Sorry Bob. I'm not doing a deal. Now you give the tablets back to Miss Jamieson and she'll give you back the six shillings. Then you take the prescription over to the chemist and get them from him. Try and do a deal with him.'

'No offance meant zir.' And he went off to the chemist. Miss Jamieson told me later that he was back again in ten minutes, money in hand, saying he would take the tablets at the price. She couldn't resist asking how much the chemist was charging and he told her nine shillings.

We had no trouble after that. Bob must have spread the word round that we were selling off the tablets at bargain price. Our reputation for moderation was never better than during the next few months.

Two events occurred during or about that time which are linked in my mind. If they are not related I shall owe an apology to the shades of Swain Galley.

As a result of my wartime experiences I was possessed for some time by a strong sense of obligation. I had had a few lucky escapes but my main war service had consisted of a long intensive post-graduate course in medicine. There was consequently no great virtue in my willingness to undertake whatever public service came my way. To begin with I went back to my weekly lectures to the St John Ambulance Brigade and joined the British Legion.

At the annual meeting of the local branch of the Legion someone proposed my name for president. I hadn't been asked beforehand and was somewhat embarrassed, because Swain Galley had held this office for some years and I hadn't the slightest wish to replace him. Moreover the president always led the Armistice parade through the town and spoke at the cenotaph the words of Laurence Binyon's 'Poem for the Fallen.' I had no relish for public appearance of that sort, but such was my mood at that time that I felt I couldn't refuse to do the job if the members wanted me to take it.

I have written about Swain Galley before and he hadn't changed during my absence. He was still a great character, an embarrassing practical joker and a local personality. Although his wife Emma had become a good friend of Jessica's I hadn't seen much of him since I attended him with erysipelas in 1938. On that occasion he had done his best to mislead me by hiding the patch of erysipelas on his leg while he tried to make me diagnose influenza. He had almost succeeded in getting me to make a fool of myself and I had been wary of him ever since. I wasn't too happy at the prospect of a direct confrontation with him over the presidency.

I sat silently in the hall while various people spoke of Swain's good service in the past and others of my own service to the community — all very embarrassing. Then someone said that after the second world war we ought to have a younger president. Swain must have been some ten or twelve years older than I was.

It happened that for some reason the chairman had to leave the meeting for a moment and, on impulse, I went over to Swain who was sitting in the front row. 'Do you want to go on doing this president's job?' I asked him.

'Depends whether they vote for me,' he said.

'If you want to carry on I won't let my name go forward in case they're misguided enough to elect me.'

'You think they'll elect you and throw me out, do you?'

He wasn't exactly a model of tact and easy converse.

'Probably not,' I answered. 'You'd rather let them vote?'

'Why not? It's a free country.'

'O.K.,' I said. If he were voted back now I should look rather small for offering to step down when his position was quite secure. It would have been more dignified to say nothing, but I had meant well. I rather hoped now that I should be elected.

The speeches went on for some time — some in favour of Swain and others for me — all polite, but a surprisingly large number of members wanted to speak. I hadn't realised at that time how many people enjoy the sound of their own voices when there is a captive audience of forty or fifty.

Finally an elderly man spoke for a full five minutes on the virtues of Swain Galley, his work for the Legion and his record of public service. This was so exaggerated that I think it must have swayed the vote in my favour.

The chairman, a good man of many years real service to the Legion, said at last that the vote must be taken and I was elected by some two votes to one. I immediately wished they had chosen Swain but was glad the voting hadn't been closer. That would have embarrassed me even more.

Swain was very polite to me after the meeting and only remarked, 'Now you'll have to get pneumonia on Armistice Day and not me.'

I thought no more about it and when Armistice Day came round I did my bit in leading the parade and speaking the words of dedication to the memory of the dead of two world wars.

It must have been several months later, though it was certainly in the cold winter that followed, that I was called out on a Sunday morning, after a heavy snowfall.

A broad Somerset voice spoke very loudly on the phone at first light — about six o'clock. 'Missus Barleymow be taken bard. She do want 'e to come over.'

'What address?' I asked.

'Zame place she's allus lived in,' said the voice, 'near the varm.'

'Which farm?'

'Monkton Varm.'

'What's the trouble?' I asked from my bed. I was waking up now.

'Er didn' zactly zay but 'er be main rough.'

'Is that her husband, Mr Barleymow?'

This seemed to be a great joke. 'Nor,' said the voice. 'Oi be a neighbour.'

'She wants me to come over now, does she?'

'Zo quick as parsible 'er did zay.'

'Alright.'

I imagined as no details were given by the male neighbour that it was probably a matter of haemorrhage — perhaps a miscarriage. It wasn't unusual for a neighbour to be called in to do the telephoning as this was regarded as a difficult procedure needing skill and experience. From a husband I might have got more information.

I dressed, took my large general purpose bag and got the car out. The snow was several inches deep and although I was able to drive up to the gate there was no doubt I should have trouble getting up the hills between here and Monkton. This meant putting on chains. There was no salt

71

on the roads and the hills could be treacherous.

Tom Wyburn and I boasted that we were never deterred by Mendip weather. Once the chains were on we would simply charge at the snowdrifts and invariably got through them. I drove back into the garage, spread out the chains and drove the car back on to them. Then I set about fixing them on. As everyone knows this is a wretched job anyway, but when your hands are frozen and the chains a tight fit it is nearly impossible. I struggled for almost half an hour, by which time I was beginning to worry lest the woman was bleeding badly. It is quite possible to die of a miscarriage.

At last I got the chains in place and bumped my way over the three miles to Monkton. There had been no traffic on the roads since the night's snowfall, but I had no trouble on the hills and made good time to the cottage. It was daylight and nearly seven when I arrived, and I expected to be greeted by an anxious husband at the door.

There was no one in sight so I knocked loudly. There was no answer. The wretched man on the phone must have given me the wrong address. Yet I knew the woman well and there was no doubt about the house unless he had given me the wrong name as well. There was only one Mrs Barleymow in Monkton.

I knocked again and at last a woman's head came out of the upstairs window.

'Mrs Barleymow,' I said, 'you sent for me. What's the trouble?'

'Tis Darcter Lane,' she gasped. 'Well I never. Wait a minute zir, I'll be down.' Then in an easily audible voice before she closed the window, 'Will, do 'e put the trousers on. Tis the darcter at the door.'

In a mintue or so the bolts were drawn, the key turned and the door opened. By this time I knew there must be a mistake. Mrs Barleymow looked at me wide-eyed. Her hair was somewhat awry but her cheeks were fresh and rosy. She looked literally in the pink of condition.

'Do 'e come in zir. Be yew in trouble on the road?'

'I'm not in trouble, no. I thought you were. Someone sent for me half an hour ago and said you were very ill.

They must have given me the wrong name. Is there anyone else ill up here? They certainly said Monkton, near the farm.'

'No zir. No one be bard up yere. Oi should know any road. They do generally zend ver me virst in a manner of speaking zir.'

I was defeated. 'Well I'm sorry to have disturbed you. There must be a mistake somewhere.'

'Can Oi get yew a cup of tea zir?'

'No thank you. I'd better get back home in case they've sent another message.'

She waited politely at her door until I was out in the road again. I waved as I got into the car where I sat for a moment thinking. Who on earth could it have been? My mind went back to the phone call. I had been asleep but I hadn't imagined it. One night before the war I had got up from a deep sleep believing I had an urgent message, and not until I was half-dressed did I realise I must have been dreaming. Jessica had heard nothing and I went back to bed too puzzled to sleep for some time. That hadn't happened this morning. The message was clear. And didn't I recognise the voice? A country voice, broader than most, with a hint of aggression in it?

Suddenly it came to me. It was Lemuel Fields, Swain Galley's man, and we were a couple of hundred yards from Swain's farm. Could it be one of his confounded practical jokes? Had Swain told Lemuel last night to phone me early this morning with a fake message, expecting to enjoy the fun when he woke up? No one had ever done such a thing before but the more I thought, the more likely did this seem. I gritted my teeth in fury. This was really going too far. And on a morning like this. I remembered the struggle I had had fixing the chains in position and vowed to get my own back somehow. In normal hours the garage would have done this for me. This was no joke at all as far as I was concerned, and it was hard to believe Swain would really be so heartless.

As I drove along to the farm on my way home the sun was just rising on a white sparkling world with the promise of a beautiful day — apart from the cold. When I drew

73

level with the farm I saw Lemuel coming out of a cowshed. Was he laughing? I couldn't quite see. 'Lem,' I shouted, 'did you telephone me an hour ago?' I knew he would be incapable of acting the joke out. He walked towards me and grinned.

I didn't smile back. 'You did, didn't you?'

'Wod ef Oi ded?' The grin was as wide as the open moorland.

'And Mr Galley told you to, didn't he?'

'Wod ef 'er ded?'

So it was Swain's doing and it wasn't a joke, it was an atrocity.

I sat in the car trying to think. The farmhouse and garden were separated from the yard and sheds by a stone wall and some trees. The yard had a separate entrance from the road and near this Swain's tractor was standing, covered with snow. It was a point of honour with Mendip farmers that they would always help a stranded motorist. I wondered whether I could somehow force Swain to come out and pull me out of trouble. Starting that tractor would be no easy job for him. Not much of a revenge but it would be something — and better than taking this lying down.

I backed through the farmhouse gateway and the next step was obvious. The roadway was on a ridge with a sharp bank on the side. If I accidentally slid down this I should certainly need a pull. I backed the car a few inches sideways and left the brake off. Gravity did the rest and the effect was to put the nearside back wheel a foot below the rest of the car. I engaged bottom gear and let in the clutch. The wheel spun and the car was well and truly stuck. I felt quite pleased with myself. It was unusual for me to think of the right reply or riposte at the right time. Almost invariably I think of the perfect answer hours after the event. This time, if the gods were with me, I could give Swain a bit of trouble in payment of my debt.

'I'm stuck, Lem. Can you give me a hand with the tractor?'

'Gaffer wun't let Oi touch tractor,' said Lem and I had expected this. Lem was a horse man. Driving a tractor was as impossible to him as flying an aeroplane. 'Oi'll give 'ee a push.'

And he pushed but even his strength was useless. To make sure he didn't get me back on the road I kept the brake on anyway. When he had pushed in vain for a minute or two I said, 'I'm afraid you'll have to get Mr Galley.'

'Er bain't up yet loike as not.'

'Then get him up. I've got to get away and don't forget I'm only here because he and you played a trick on me.'

The reminder of this brought a smile back to Lem's sweating face and he went off to the back door of the house.

I waited a full five minutes. Swain was taking his time. Perhaps I had put myself too much in his power. I hadn't thought my plan through properly. Presently I saw Lem walking across the yard towards the sheds, so I went down the garden by the wall and called after him.

'Gaffer reckoned 'e'll be out prenly,' he said.

I waited another five minutes and got very cold. My splendid plan had backfired badly and I had only made matters worse for myself. I approached Lem again and this time heard the worst.

'Did you tell Mr Galley I'm stuck in the snow?' I asked him.

'Ah. Arf an hour 'er zaid.'

'Half an hour! I can't hang about like that.' Annoyed with myself now I took my bag out and then locked the car. I knew if I could have got hold of Emma, Swain's wife, she would have insisted on his coming out at once, but there was no way of making contact with her without Swain blocking the way. I had had enough indignity for one cold morning and strode off to the telephone box in the middle of the village. I phoned the garage and asked for help. I needed a lift home. I knew I could rely on help from them at any hour of the day or night. I had delivered the owner's wife of their first baby early in the war and only got him breathing with difficulty. There was nothing special about this but they always behaved as though they owed me a great deal, and I benefited from many years of extreme kindness from that family. I soon had the promise of an immediate rescue.

I didn't want to meet Swain Galley now and set off

towards Melbrook. As I walked along through the snow a small consolation struck me. My car was completely blocking the Galleys' drive. No one could get in or out through it. Remembering the long minutes I had waited with no response whatever from Swain this gave me some satisfaction. What was more, he couldn't move my car because it was well and truly locked with the hand-brake on. No tractor could pull it up that slope without my cooperation. In due course I was met by the car from the garage. My rescuer offered to pull my car out of its trouble but I told him I preferred to leave it where it was for the present.

'Swain won't be pleased,' he said.

'I don't intend him to be.' And before long I was telling the tale over a hot breakfast.

All I had to do now was to wait — unless another urgent message came in. Then I should have to borrow a car from the garage but even this was worthwhile.

Time passed and I began to wonder whether Swain was prepared to leave his drive blocked indefinitely. It was two hours later that the phone call came. Swain wanted to get out of his drive and my car was blocking the way.

'Oh,' I said. 'I'm sorry. You were so long coming out that I couldn't wait. You'll have to come and fetch me I'm afraid. I have no other car.'

'But I can't get out,' he shouted.

'Too bad,' I replied. 'Well, if you send someone down I'll come up and steer the car while you give me a pull with the tractor.'

There was silence at the other end and I asked, 'Well Swain?'

'You drove it down there on purpose, didn't you?'

'Whatever makes you say that?'

'Alright, you stay there and I'll send someone down.'

'I can't promise to be here. I'll do my best but if anything urgent comes in I may have to let myself be fetched to do the call.'

What he said then was not couched in terms fit to write down in a record of this sort, but in due course a neighbour of his arrived and drove me back to Monkton. A few minutes later my car was back on the road again.

'Thanks for the pull, Swain,' I said. 'And thanks for getting Lem to phone me about Mrs Barleymow at six o'clock.'

'What makes you think I told him to?'

He turned his back on me and walked with his heavy stride back through the gate to the farmhouse. I think it was fair to admit that he had got the better of me and that we had both behaved like schoolboys, but anyway he never played the same trick on me again.

7

Family doctors work for a long time to attain a position of trust and this very trust becomes their most valuable therapeutic weapon. The advances in medical knowledge provided my generation with a great deal of help in this direction. We were the lucky ones who were first handed the powerful and dramatic new drugs of penicillin and sulphonamide by which we were able, at a stroke, to annihilate the horrors of many ancient nightmares. Naturally after this our patients were more ready to trust us.

The stories I have told in the past relate to the steps by which I worked my way from the newly qualified to the more experienced and accepted general practitioner. The second stage of what is called experience is unending because it consists of learning about people. The effect of mind on body, of emotion in the production of physical disease, renders this area of experience essential to medical practice. Fortunately it is as fascinating as it is important.

With its love of impressive-sounding Greek words, our profession soon admitted the truth of the dependence of body on mind by announcing that certain diseases were psychosomatic. Psychiatry had been taught for a century but it didn't seem to help us much in treating the day to day sicknesses of ordinary people. It was with almost infinite slowness that the idea spread that feelings, emotions, relationships played a real part in the production of common diseases. At the same time many of us were beginning to realise that we knew pathetically little about real people.

Soon after the war I had one of my first lessons in

understanding people, and this was that I knew very little about them.

Susie Bordon was a rather angular woman with pointed elbows and knees that are said to indicate a shrewish temper. She had a prominent but straight and pointed nose that seemed to quiver with curiosity when she was engaged in her favourite occupation of studying other people's business. She gathered information as a frugal mother gathers stores for her family.

'Nothing human comes amiss to me' was a motto instilled into me years ago by my father, but I have to confess that my hackles rose whenever Susie came to see me. Any reaction of that sort is of course the shortest cut in existence to bad diagnosis. You are apt to listen unsympathetically and ignore danger signals which would normally set the alarm bells ringing.

One of Susie's sources of information was the surgery. She would arrive long before the time of her appointment and then, according to my watchful receptionist, she would make a study of the other patients, somehow getting them to tell her all about their problems and their ailments.

Her method with me would have been entertaining if I had not lost my sense of humour as soon as she came into the room. 'Poor Mrs Brown's been in to see you, hasn't she?' she would say, 'it's her back again isn't it?'

I would smile non-committally, believing that even my silence would give away something profoundly confidential to this piece of absorbent sponge.

Then she would go on, 'She told me it was making her life a misery. So much pain. Day after day. I think her husband is a lot of the trouble. He's so mean. He could easily afford to buy her a washing-machine but she has to do every bit of her laundry in the bath, bending over it for hours scrubbing those children's things. But there's nothing seriously wrong with her, is there?'

She would wait for some response from me and I would sidestep as well as I could and bring the conversation back to her affairs.

One day she came to see me with a rash on her hands and

arms. It seemed likely to be an allergy to one of the detergent powders and was fairly quickly dealt with. Before she left she spoke of Dinah Barrett whose wedding had been postponed because of her illness.

'Poor Dinah,' she said. 'Isn't it sad? Such a lovely girl too.'

I nodded and smiled my sympathy.

'My heart bleeds for that lovely young man too,' Susie went on. 'Mmm.' Her mind seemed to be dwelling on the passionate union that had been postponed.

I murmured something intended to be both sympathetic and dismissive, but Susie's desire for an emotional orgy was not to be denied.

'That tuberculosis is such an awful disease, Doctor. One of my neighbours had it as you know and the cough was terrible to listen to.'

'Let's hope Dinah will soon improve,' I said.

'Oh so you think it's been taken early then? Can you cure it if it's taken early enough?'

'It's quite possible.' I stressed the last word and moved to the door to open it for her. This sort of interrogation always annoyed me because it presented one with the dilemma of either being rude or saying something that could be misconstrued and quoted in a way that gave the impression of a breach of confidence.

Susie was harder to move than ever that day. 'Is it very infections — tuberculosis?'

'It is infectious but only by fairly long and close contact.'

'Mrs Barrett is looking for help in the house and she's asked me if I would give her three mornings a week, but with my family I don't think I could. I mean if I caught it what would happen to Ben and Doreen?' These were her two children.

'There would be very little risk of catching it like that, even if Dinah were staying at home.'

'She's going to hospital then?'

'Yes.'

'But there's some risk, you would say?'

She was asking me the impossible. I couldn't deny there

was some small element of risk to domestic staff working in the house where someone had active tuberculosis, though in this case it was minimal. 'A very small risk,' I said, 'less than, shall we say, driving a car. Let me see you at the end of the week if your hands don't improve.'

But Susie wasn't ready to leave yet. 'I wonder where poor Dinah caught it from. From some patient when she was working in the hospital in London, I suppose.'

'Possibly.'

'And she wouldn't have been very close to the patients, would she? I mean nurses aren't bending over their patients all the time, are they?'

'No, of course not.'

'So if she caught it from a patient she only saw a few times I might catch it from her the same, mightn't I?'

By this time I was becoming thoroughly irritated. Thinking about the interview afterwards I realised that she was only putting questions to me that she had every right to ask, but at the same time it seemed that I was being forced to break confidence. 'Now will you ask Miss Jamieson to send in the next patient,' I said and at last she went.

I sighed with relief. It was seldom that the trick of holding the door open failed to make a patient take the hint and I only used it rarely. I felt as though I had been cross-examined by a skilful barrister who was bent on ruining my reputation.

Perhaps I was unduly fussy about confidentiality, but a great deal in medical practice depends on your patients being absolutely certain that their affairs will never be divulged by their doctor without their consent. Tom Wyburn was perhaps too rigid in his application of the Hippocratic principles and he had been drumming his ideas into me for years. If you are innocently asked a question about a patient and refuse to answer it, it is easy to give a false and harmful impression. For instance, suppose an employer suspected one of his staff of having V.D. and asked a direct question about it. If the person concerned was not suffering from V.D. it would be wrong to say 'I can't discuss his affairs with you' because this would suggest that he was.

The problem is never easy and occasionally bothered me. As a result I was sometimes annoyed by quite innocent questions.

I went to see Dinah Barrett a day or two later. She was still waiting for a hospital bed. On the landing upstairs I noticed a woman cleaning and said casually to Mrs Barrett, 'I see you've got some help. I'm glad of that. You need it.'

Dinah was looking remarkably well, sitting up in bed in a large room overlooking the garden. When we had finished our consultation which at the moment consisted of a chat about plans for the future, her mother told me I had done her a service over the domestic help. 'I had engaged Mrs Bordon — a patient of yours — but she came to see me saying you had advised her not to come here as she might catch Dinah's trouble.' She was laughing as she spoke but I gasped.

'I never did anything of the sort,' I said defensively. 'She is the most impossible woman. She kept nagging me to say there was no risk whatever in contact with a tuberculous patient, and no one in their senses could guarantee that. There is of course some small degree of risk to susceptible people. But believe me, I never said anything definite like that. She's a dangerous woman. Perhaps you are better off without her.'

Mrs Barrett laughed at my fury. 'Don't worry. I knew you wouldn't say anything to embarrass us. But you see you did us a good turn. You saved me from having to tell her that I had changed my mind. The woman I found after I had engaged Mrs Bordon is much more suitable, and such a dear. I didn't know how I was going to tell her.'

I shook my head and changed the subject.

On my way home I started wondering what to do about Susie Bordon. She had forced me to admit a small degree of risk to a domestic worker at the Barretts and then twisted my admission into direct advice to stay away. I knew well enough that this was how patients often used what we said, but it was embarrassing all the same. A less understanding woman than Mrs Barrett might have been justifiably angry. I began to think seriously of having

Susie removed from my list, but as soon as my attention was taken up by other patients I let the matter slide.

Within the next few weeks I was faced with one of those tragedies that tend to shatter your faith in the essential goodness of the universe and it was then that Susie's activities reached a climax.

I was sent for by a young Pole who went by the anglicised name of Bluejack. He was a single man living in lodgings with a family I will call Smithers. He was a pleasant fellow, kindly, sensitive and warm-hearted, and a good worker in the factory where he had gained in responsibility till he had become a charge hand. There was no urgency about the message and it was mid-afternoon on a late summer day that I visited him. The house was in one of the new estates, well kept and furnished, and spotlessly clean. Bluejack lived with the family and occupied the fourth bedroom, overlooking a farm and open fields to the west where the ground rose gently to the Mendips. Mrs Smithers was a small neat woman, usually placid but that day obviously worried. 'He's lost the use of his legs,' she said. 'I hope it's not a stroke.' As Bluejack was only just over thirty this seemed unlikely.

His face was round, ruddy and remarkably cheerful for someone in serious trouble. I was more concerned than he was at what I found. There was gross weakness of his legs but normal sensation, and I thought at first he must have contracted poliomyelitis — infantile paralysis is an unsatisfactory name for a disease in middle life. When I asked him about his recent health, thinking he might have had a feverish attack leading up to his present trouble, he told me that a few months ago he had partly lost the sight of one eye for a time but as it had got better quickly he had not bothered me about it. When I examined his eyes there was evidence of what had caused his temporary loss of vision, and this with the signs in his legs pretty well clinched the diagnosis. It was almost certain that he had multiple sclerosis.

In hospital this might have caused a degree of not unpleasant excitement in the house physician. It was a definite 'case'. But in country practice it was a tragedy.

I told Bluejack that he would probably recover much of the use of his legs in a week or two and that I would have him examined by a neurologist in the city hospital. In due course the specialist agreed the diagnosis and there was some improvement in the weakness of his legs, but his future prospects were grim. Multiple sclerosis can affect any part of the nervous system and there is only partial recovery from each of its ravages. Further attacks may strike at any time, perhaps in weeks, perhaps not for years. It plays with its victim like a cat with a mouse.

In spite of some improvement we had to get him an invalid chair — provided before the introduction of the National Health Service by the Red Cross. He was a determined character and confident of his recovery. He soon managed to get down the stairs by sitting on each one and sliding down to the next, then scrambled into his chair at the bottom.

Mrs Smithers was faced with a dilemma. She went out to work herself and the children were at school. Her husband was rather a rigid and exacting character and in a few weeks the extra burden of Bluejack's illness began to tell on her. For a time he was partially incontinent and this was the last straw. One day she came to see me saying that he would have to go.

'Couldn't he go into hospital?' she asked.

I shook my head. The cottage hospital still only accepted surgical patients and anyway a chronic case was out of the question. It would block a bed intended for acute surgery. The only alternative was a chronic sick bed usually kept for old people and these were nearly always full. Bluejack was neither old nor permanently sick. In time he should improve enough to go back to work provided he had no further attacks.

I sympathised with Mrs Smithers. She could foresee keeping a chronic invalid in the house for months ahead. Her husband was pressing her to get rid of Bluejack and the tension in the house was rising day by day.

My own main sympathy, however, was with Bluejack. Life in a chronic sick hospital at that time was utterly bleak. The beds were still in the former workhouse buildings and were occupied by old people in various stages of mental and physical decay. To put a young man with a keen, sensitive, and active brain into such surroundings was unthinkable. He might be imprisoned there for twenty or thirty years. Real prison would be infinitely preferable.

I telephoned the relieving officer but he could offer nothing but a bed in the workhouse four miles away, and the case settled on my mind as an unsolved problem that nagged incessantly.

One day I came across a man in a wheelchair working his way laboriously along the pavement by turning the wheels with his hands. It was Bluejack. I stopped the car alongside. 'Where are you off to?' I asked.

'I'm going down to the factory. I want to see if they'll have me back. I could do my own job if they'll let me use the chair.'

'You feel up to it?'

'I feel alright. It's just my legs. This other trouble — the waterworks — that's better.'

'You're a charge hand, aren't you?'

'Yes, but I don't care what I do if they'll give me something. It's not the money. It's being some use in the world.'

I wished him luck but even a job didn't solve the problem of where he could live. I couldn't help admiring him. He was cheerful even under this burden. I hadn't discussed his future with him and he was obviously expecting to recover in a few weeks. Time enough to talk about the future when he had another attack.

That same afternoon he turned up at the surgery. The factory manager had agreed to let him try his own job, getting about in his chair, so I gave him a signing-off note. So far, so good, but what about Mrs Smithers? I hoped she would agree to keep him now that he was going back to work, but I reckoned without her husband. He came to see me a day or two later and quickly put his point of view.

'This disease,' he said, 'this multiple sclerosis, I've been looking it up in the Doctor's Book. It leads to paralysis, doesn't it? Gets steadily worse. Well we can't possibly keep him in our house. The wife's already getting worn out with all this laundry and whatnot. He'll have to go.'

'He's not incontinent now, is he? And he gets about almost normally in his chair.'

'That's not the point. It's the future I'm worried about. What's going to happen when he gets paralysed and stuck in bed all the time? We couldn't turn him out into the streets like that. He'll have to go now.'

I couldn't deny the possibilities. 'It might be years before he gets another attack,' I said, 'possibly never. And if you insist on moving him it means a bed in a chronic sick hospital and no chance of work. Could you keep him for a time while he tries to find somewhere else? If the worst came to the worst and he became paralysed, we should get him into hospital straight away. You certainly wouldn't be burdened with him.'

'We can't keep him for long. I've told him he'll have to go. I'm sorry for the chap but we've got ourselves to consider. Would you have him in your house with young children to look after?'

'If he were already there I don't think I could turn him out, but I see your problem. Will you wait a week or two while we try to find him somewhere else?'

Unwillingly he agreed. It was impossible for poor Bluejack to go round in a wheelchair asking for someone to take him in, so I was left with the problem. Welfare services, compared with what they became under the N.H.S., were virtually nonexistent at that time and there was no official help available. With the spectre of Bluejack fretting out his days in the squalid smelly wards occupied by the old and dying, I doubled my efforts to find him a home. I asked the help of the vicar, the Women's Institute, the Red Cross, the nonconformist churches and the British Legion, but I knew it was asking a great deal to expect a family to take in a stranger whose prospects included paralysis, and worse, within a few years. Was there any good Samaritan who would give him a home? At that time he would be little trouble and there was always a chance that he would suffer no deterioration. A week passed and there appeared no hope.

Mr Smithers came to see me again and told me he had given Bluejack a week's notice.

Then Bluejack came to see me again. His cheerful ruddy face was not unduly worried even now. He had improved enough to do a good deal more without his chair. Obviously he didn't know anything about the grisly prospects of his disease and I was determined not to enlighten him.

'I've been given notice,' he said, 'by Mr Smithers.'

'I was afraid that was coming. Mr Smithers came to see me.'

'I'm much better now but it's the future that worries them. They've been reading about my case in the Doctor's Book. I'd found out about it myself too but I wasn't going to say anything. Most people with this thing end up as invalids, so I can't blame them. I want to work as long as I can.'

So he knew all about it.

'If you've read about it you know that you may never get any more trouble, or it may be many years before you do.'

He smiled ruefully. Courage, real courage, has always moved me profoundly, and here it was. 'You're trying to cheer me up,' he said. 'I came to ask about something I've heard. There's a community like a monastery down at Cerne Abbas. A friend of mine thought I might get in there.'

The idea was new to me and brought a ray of hope, but it would take him away from his work at the factory. We agreed that he and I should both write to Cerne Abbas but I should go on trying to find a home for him in the district.

Today an army of welfare workers would take all this worry off the doctor's shoulders. In fact he would never be conscious of anxiety on the patient's behalf, because the patient's accommodation is not his responsibility. In 1946 it was very much his problem.

Another week passed and I was beginning to give up hope that any family would offer a home to a partially paralysed foreigner with a prospect of complete invalidism in the future. The prospect of a chronic sick bed loomed nearer. The British Legion would give him two weeks holiday in one of their homes but this would solve nothing. The thought of sending him to a chronic sick ward with all its hopeless faces, the bent staggering figures, the smells, the gradually emptying beds as one prisoner and then another was released from the ward by death, looked like becoming a reality.

I called at various houses where I knew apartments had been let in the past, but for one reason or another none could take him.

Then to increase my concern about Bluejack, Susie Bordon came to see me with some triviality and insisted on discussing his case. She seemed to be longing to indulge in an orgy of sympathy and when she began to ask about his future I shut up like a clam. I wasn't going to satisfy this woman's emotional wallowings for anyone.

'An awful disease this multiple sclerosis, isn't it?' she said. 'I heard of a case once. Incontinent she was poor thing. What will happen to Mr Bluejack?'

'It's impossible to tell,' I told her. 'What he needs is a home to live in.'

'Suppose he became incontinent?' she asked.

'Well?' I said brusquely.

'It would be terrible for him. And for anyone he lived with too. Such a lot of work.'

I couldn't stand any more. I handed her a prescription and walked silently to the door and opened it for her. This time there was a hint of reproach in her expression as she left.

She was the last patient that evening and I spoke to Miss Jamieson as soon as the door closed behind her. 'That woman,' I said. 'That woman.'

'You don't seem to like her. She's quite kind-hearted really.'

'Now why do you say that? She's determined to find out every detail of every other patient's troubles, including diagnosis, prognosis and treatment. There's nothing very kind about that.'

Miss Jamieson smiled. 'Perhaps she's sorry for them.'

Annabel Jamieson, I thought to myself, is quite a decent soul but she's no judge of character. She doesn't know this woman as I do.

A few days later I had a letter marked 'confidential'

which had therefore been left unopened on my desk.

It was headed with Susie Bordon's address and for a moment the thought struck me that I had offended her and that she was asking to be removed from my list of patients. This was unusual and very polite of her because in the days before the N.H.S., private patients left you without a word if they wanted to change their doctor and Susie came under the heading of private patients. All the better, I thought. Then, reading on, words of real gratitude puzzled me. 'No one else would have been so kind — you have been more than a doctor — more than a friend —' And now apparently all my efforts had been rewarded.

Puzzled, I glanced down at the signature. It was signed M. Bluejack.

Mrs Bordon had taken him into her home and welcomed him as one of her family.

I sat back staring at the letter and then at my own misjudgement. It was almost unbelievable. Susie had been asking about Bluejack's future because she was making up her mind to give him a home. When, oh God, when should I begin to understand the complexities of human nature?

I talked to Jessica about the affair that evening and she reminded me of two lines of Robbie Burns.

'Then gently scan your brother man
Still gentlier sister woman.'

'That's all very well, but this woman seemed to spend all her time finding out about other people. Annabel Jamieson said she was just sorry for them but I didn't believe it.'

'You've only told me about her twice. The other time was when she asked whether there was any risk of catching TB from Dinah Barrett. That was a fair question if she was thinking of going to work there.'

'I suppose it was but —' I hated admitting how wrong I had been. Preconceived ideas about people's characters' could be very powerful and very mistaken. 'And her pointed nose,' I said lamely. 'And her pointed elbows and scraggy knees.'

'What have they got to do with her character? If you talk to a cripple you needn't look at his feet.'

'Too subtle,' I said.

'You can't judge people's characters by what they look like. You wear glasses but that doesn't mean you are feeble. She can't help her pointed nose. She's obviously a very generous and kind-hearted woman.'

'O.K., O.K. It's easy for you because you know the end of the story.' I also knew that her first impressions were more reliable than mine.

Bluejack stayed with the Bordons for years and became one of the family. Eventually his condition deteriorated but he never lacked a family or friends. If ever my faith in human nature begins to falter I think of Susie. And how right you were, Robbie Burns.

Knowing that I had been quite wrong about Susie Bordon troubled me for a time. I was forty years old and ought to have been a shrewd judge of character. Naturally I saw her with different eyes after this. When she asked about one of my patients I realised that it was not necessarily from idle curiosity. She was possessed of enormous compassion and wanted to help everyone in the world.

The most curious thing of all was that her pointed nose, which had seemed to quiver with curiosity, looked different. She became gentle and warm-hearted. Thinking about the changes in her, it was clear that it was I who had changed. I suppose it was then that I began to understand that every interview with a patient is a two-way affair. If you showed disapproval or dislike or any sort of prejudice the patient's manner would change, and a vicious circle of mutual antagonism would develop.

The doctor in his consulting-room is not the great 'I AM'. He changes, like everyone else, in response to the presence of other people. It is necessary, particularly in our work, to study our own reactions as well as the patient's.

8

It was on the day I fell into the stinging nettles that I was first called to see Miss Maynard. The two events are associated in my mind because they have something in common. The one gave me a few hours of irritation over the upper half of my body and the case of Miss Maynard caused me some weeks of perplexity.

One summer afternoon I was in the garden picking some of the early Tom Putt apples. I was stripped to the waist like the children and balancing on top of a rickety pair of steps when the thing toppled over and threw me into an angry, lush, three-foot-high bed of nettles. The children were kindly young folk but the sight of Father diving headlong into the worst bed of nettles in England was too much for them. They literally roared with laughter.

While my wife was giving first aid to my outraged back the telephone rang. The message was urgent. Miss Maynard's maid said at some length that her mistress was apparently unconscious. She was sitting in her chair staring in front of her and making small grunting noises. And she was deadly pale. I dressed as quickly as I could and hurried off to the village some four miles away where she lived. She was a newcomer to the district and I hadn't seen her before.

The house, on the outskirts of Rock Weston, was a large one for two people. The entrance was quite imposing and at the side of the house. It gave the visitor a good view of the garden while he waited to be admitted. The garden itself must have covered about an acre and, as I discovered later, was looked after by a full-time gardener. There was a large lawn behind the house with a fifty-foot rose bed on one side and well-established shrubs on the other. At first glance there was not a weed in the place.

Inside, the house was one of those obsessively tidy places that make you expect an occupant of rigid habit and character — a description that certainly didn't apply to Miss Maynard.

I was shown into a small room evidently used as a sewing-room and found Miss Maynard sitting by the open window enjoying the sunshine. The first disconcerting thing about the interview was that she thought I was the man who had come to read the gas meter. I explained who I was and that her maid had sent for me because she thought she was ill. This puzzled her and she politely denied any possibility of illness. 'Whatever made Elsa think that,' she said. 'I've never felt better. I did my usual walk in the garden this morning, ate my usual lunch — brown bread, cheddar cheese and an apple — then came in here to rest. Sometimes I shut my eyes in the afternoon and sometimes I don't.'

She beamed at me, apologised for my being troubled and obviously expected me to leave, but the maid must have had some reason for calling me and I persevered with what was ostensibly a social chat. I gathered that her father had been a 'businessman' and in her early years she had done some missionary work. For ten years now she had been retired and lived with Elsa Dowry, her maid, who was a woman of about her own age.

I asked if she had chosen Somerset for any special reason and she said she had always wanted to come south from the Midlands. She had seen a notice in *Country Life* advertising her present house, had come to see it, liked it and bought it six months ago. She was keen on gardening and cats — of whom I saw three at my first visit. All perfectly normal and I was left puzzling over the maid's urgent message.

'So kind of you to call and see me,' said Miss Maynard. 'If I need a doctor I shall know who to send for. Thank you so much.'

As I prepared to leave she said 'Everyone has been very

kind to me here.' She laughed and added, 'A little too kind. There's one thing that puzzles me — a strange man calls on me every Thursday. He always expects tea and says he can't drink Indian tea and prefers Earl Grey. Such a strange man. I can't think why he comes to see us.'

This sounded very odd. Was she a little mentally confused? Surely she wouldn't give tea to a strange man every Thursday without having the least idea who he was. And special tea too.

'A local man?' I asked.

'He must be. You must think it strange of me not to know who he is, but the first time he came he told us he was a neighbour and he hoped we had settled in comfortably. Very polite of him. Then he came again and I didn't like to ask why he had come. I don't even know his name. And now every time he comes it is more difficult to ask him who he is.' She laughed quite cheerfully and I accepted that she had been led into an embarrassing situation that might afflict anyone.

My impression of her was a pleasant one. She was a nice old lady with charming manners. I was still puzzled about the reason for my being called. The maid must have been deceived in some way. Perhaps a few words with her would elucidate matters.

'Miss Maynard seems very well now,' I said to the maid. 'Tell me what she was like when you sent for me. You thought she was unconscious? Were her eyes closed?'

'No. They were wide open as though she was staring at something I couldn't see. And she looked deadly pale — as though she had seen a ghost.' Elsa looked frightened.

'Did you talk to her?'

'She wouldn't answer me. I stood straight in front of her and said Miss Maynard, Miss Maynard. And she looked right through me. I was scared, I can tell you.'

'Has she ever been like that before?'

'No, never. Sometimes she is a bit forgetful but never like that.'

'Who is the man who comes to see her every Thursday and stays to tea? Do you know him?'

She looked at a loss. 'No one comes to tea on Thursdays

nor any other days — except the vicar. He's been about twice.'

'So you think she's imagining this man?'

'No one comes, I can tell you that.' She looked stubborn and aggressive when I would have expected her to be puzzled and worried. Evidently she wanted to protect her mistress from undue enquiries.

I talked to her for some minutes while I adjusted my ideas about Miss Maynard. She might be subject to hallucinations. If so I couldn't guess at the cause of them unless they were presenile, and she shewed no other signs of premature aging. On the other hand she might have had a minor attack of epilepsy which could cause her to stare into space. This might cause temporary confusion but if so her mind would clear in a short while. She certainly hadn't appeared to be in a post-epileptic state.

The maid's manner was odd, as though she knew more than she was telling me, but I could get nothing more out of her. The question now was whether or not I ought to see the mistress again. If she was mentally ill I ought to keep in touch with her, and if she had had a first attack of epilepsy she would need investigation. I decided to see her again in a few days and said so to the maid.

The queer thing was that of the two of them the maid seemed more abnormal than the mistress, not by what she said but by her manner of saying it. Anyway here was an apparently harmless old lady, suffering either from presenile hallucinations or from minor epilepsy, who needed to be kept under observation.

As I left, my assessment of the situation was suddenly shattered. 'The only man who comes to see us,' said the maid, 'is Miss Maynard's father.'

'Her father?' Miss Maynard must have been in her seventies and her father would be at least in his nineties. It was very odd that someone of that age should be calling on his daughter. 'Where does he live then — Miss Maynard's father?'

'Oh I don't know where he lives now.'

'He doesn't live here in Rock Weston then?'

'No, no. He doesn't live anywhere near here.'

94

'Then how does he get here?'

'It's not my place to ask that. He comes about once a month. You never know when he's coming. He just arrives in time for lunch with Miss Maynard.'

Now I was really puzzled. The maid seemed to be the one who was unbalanced, and if so there might be a genuine dropper-in who came to tea on Thursdays. It was easier to believe this than that the old lady's father came to lunch every month — unless he was a very well-preserved old gentleman indeed.

I couldn't leave the matter there so I went back to see the mistress. Elsa showed no inclination to follow me. She stayed in the kitchen while I went back to the sewing-room and closed the door.

'Forgive me for coming back, Miss Maynard,' I said, 'but I'm rather puzzled. May I ask you whether your father is still alive?'

'My father? What makes you ask that? No of course not. My father died years ago.'

'To be perfectly frank it is your maid who puzzles me. She told me that your father comes to lunch every month or so. Does she get confused?'

'Oh, Elsa is a little strange sometimes, but she is so good and I couldn't manage without her.' She smiled benignly again. I would have expected her to be at least embarrassed and probably upset by the news that she was living with someone completely divorced from reality.

'She evidently sent for me because she imagined you were ill this afternoon?'

'Quite likely. Quite likely.' She laughed again as cheerfully as ever. 'Don't take any notice of Elsa. I'll telephone you myself if I want you.'

'I think, if you don't mind, I would like to call again to see your maid. She does seem to be confused — mentally unbalanced in fact. First she said you were unconscious and she couldn't rouse you, and now she says you never have a guest on Thursdays whereas you tell me that a man comes to see you regularly.'

'She is a little strange. But don't worry. I understand her.' She beamed at me again. Clearly it was the maid and not the mistress who was confused. At least I had settled that problem.

'Your stranger — he wasn't the vicar by any chance?'

'Oh no, not the vicar dressed like that.' She laughed again. 'He wears such funny clothes. He's rather — shall we say well-built — and he wears a bright red jersey that is very tight on his stomach and a green and white striped cap that he seems very proud of. Mustn't forget my cap, he says when he leaves me.' Her laughter sounded merry and unworried but I was once more plunged into an abyss of uncertainty.

I pictured a sort of Tweedledum in bright red jersey and green and white striped cap — an outfit surely no ordinary person would wear to call on an elderly lady who was a complete stranger. Was she too —? But this was getting ridiculous. She looked so charming and so utterly normal. I felt I really must get away before I began to doubt my own sanity.

That evening I tried to work out the evidence of mental confusion in the two ladies. When I told Jessica about it she found my story difficult to believe. She even wondered whether the large dose of nettle stings I was still suffering from had made me lose my sense of proportion.

The facts were something like this. Miss Maynard had appeared to be in a trance and this was the reason for my being sent for. She might have been in some catatonic or possibly epileptic state, or on the other hand the maid might have imagined it. No good.

There was the stranger who came to tea on Thursdays. He might have been a genuine stranger but why so oddly dressed? Was there really a local character who dressed up like Tweedledum in the illustrations of the Alice books and went out to tea demanding no other than Earl Grey tea? A very unlikely story, but if there were such a person and Elsa the maid denied his existence then Elsa was unbalanced. If not, it was the mistress.

The visits of Miss Maynard's father related by the maid and denied by the mistress almost certainly indicated illusions on the part of the maid. If the maid was abnormal you couldn't rely on what she said about the mistress.

It seemed as though both the old ladies were suffering from some degree of mental disturbance. I could accept that the maid was unbalanced but it was hard to believe that the mistress was anything other than a very nice old lady. It was like a Chinese puzzle but I really had to make up my mind. I thought of the play *Arsenic and Old Lace*. The most terrible things might happen and I should be responsible.

I had one hope of help and that was from Annabel Jamieson. She lived in Rock Weston and would certainly know what the village people thought of the two ladies. I talked to her on Monday morning.

'Do you have any strange characters living out at Rock Weston?'

She laughed and said she supposed there were a few oddities.

'Do you know a Miss Elsa Dowry, maid to Miss Maynard?'

'Yes, I've seen her about. Rather a silent person. She doesn't talk much but that's all to the good in the village shop!'

'Is she regarded as quite normal — mentally normal I mean?'

Annabel looked at me in surprise. 'Yes, I think so. I'm sure I should have heard if there were anything queer about her.'

'Try and find out what they think of her in the village shop and the post office.'

'I'll do my best. I'm not much good at being Sherlock Holmes but I'll try.'

Then I told her about my visit to the Maynard house on Saturday afternoon and got her intrigued by the problem. 'I'm sure the maid must be normal,' Annabel said. 'People would have noticed if she weren't. It must be the mistress who is mental. I've never seen her about.'

'You may be right. She tells me that a man dressed in a bright red sweater and a green and white striped cap goes to tea with her every Thursday, demands Earl Grey tea, and she doesn't even know who he is. He sounds like the illustrations of Tweedledum.'

This made her laugh. 'Oh well it's obvious, isn't it? There are no Tweedledums or Tweedledees in Weston. She must be imagining it.'

During the next few days Annabel brought me a little more information. Miss Dowry was said by the owner of the village shop to be very quiet but a good customer. She always paid on the spot, asked no questions, never talked about her mistress or her work or her past life. She went to the shop every Tuesday and Friday, bought her things, paid cash for them and spoke to no one else. 'Not very friendly but quite a nice woman' was the verdict of the shop, which meant Mrs Peart who was a shrewd character.

'No sign of Tweedledum?' I asked.

'None whatever.'

'And no visiting nonagenarians?'

'No.'

I began to doubt Miss Maynard's mental balance again. If Elsa had been abnormal the village people would surely have spotted it. Country people are shrewd observers of human character. Their instinct for diagnosing mental illness is usually very sound. The pendulum swung once more in favour of Elsa being the normal one.

One sure way of settling the matter was to call on Miss Maynard on Thursday at teatime and see for myself whether the curious visitor materialised. On the other hand, Thursday was my precious half-day and before the era of television, Jessica and I used to go fairly regularly to Bath on that day, do some shopping, have tea at Forts restaurant and go to the pictures. On summer days we would go for a long walk, but in either case those few hours represented our only escape in the week from the practice. I was reluctant to give this up for anything that was not really urgent. As it was, we were caught often enough just as we were leaving home by a call from someone who wanted me personally or by a maternity case which took priority over all else.

The summer I am writing about was 1947 and it was not until the end of that year that Tom Wyburn and I took the advanced step of taking alternate weekends off. This meant we would take no new messages from noon on Saturday until ten o'clock on Sunday evening. We would still do our routine visits during the weekend and any maternity cases that came along, but often we would have twenty-four hours of freedom. This glorious advance however was some months ahead of us, so I didn't call on Miss Maynard on a Thursday afternoon.

I talked to Tom Wyburn about the problem and he offered to help. 'Would you like me to call on Thursday?' he asked. 'It might look a bit strange but it would solve your dilemma.'

'No, of course not. We shall have to wait and see what happens. Besides Tweedledum might not turn up that day. Then we should be none the wiser.'

'But if he did turn up,' said Wyburn solemnly, 'what a triumph! I must say I should be fascinated to see him. Do you think he wears striped shorts as well?' By this time he was as intrigued as I was.

'It's a crazy situation,' I said. 'The best thing I can do is to forget about it.'

I did however call on the Friday of that week — feeling more like a detective than a doctor. The only hope of clearing the case up was by talking to Miss Maynard herself. I was as frank with her as possible, hoping she would give herself away, but before long her complete normality impressed itself on me once more.

'I'm still a little concerned about your maid,' I remarked. 'She seems to suffer from these extraordinary hallucinations.'

'Oh dear, these long words. You mean she imagines things?'

'Yes. I told you she said your father came to lunch with you every month. Then she denied that anyone came to tea with you when in fact you told me you had a regular visitor. What do you make of it?'

She looked serious for a moment. 'Yes I know she is a little strange, but that does no harm does it? I think really she is a little jealous of someone coming to see me, so she pretends no one comes. Can you understand that? As to my father, are you sure you didn't misunderstand her?'

'No, I don't think so. But you find her entirely satisfactory? She never upsets you in any way?'

'No. She's very good. No one is perfect and sometimes she sulks a little but I just wait till she gets over it and all is well.' The bright smile came again and I found I was liking her more and more. I was sure now that there was nothing mentally wrong with her. I would have liked to solve the Tweedledum problem but there was nothing more I could do about it.

Several weeks later I called once more, but both ladies were then equally on the defensive. Elsa was markedly hostile and my conversations with her in passing were completely sterile. Miss Maynard herself, though still polite, seemed to be resisting any further investigation on my part. She was not ill, she said. She had had no further unconscious attacks suggesting epilepsy. She was well aware that Elsa was 'a little strange' but had no wish to pursue the matter any further. I felt she would prefer me to mind my own business but was too polite to say so. I decided not to call any more unless I was sent for. There might be some explanation of the strangely-clad Thursday visitor but unless it materialised I should have to keep an open mind.

There my interest in the case would have had to end but for Annabel Jamieson. She greeted me one morning with suppressed excitement. 'I've seen your Tweedledum,' she whispered to me before surgery. When she was excited she opened her eyes very wide and spoke very quietly.

She came into my room and closed the door. 'He's a retired schoolmaster in Rock Weston,' she said. 'He came to live with his daughter about a year ago. I'd seen him about in the village but never in the red jersey and green cap. Yesterday he was! Not like Tweedledum but with a jacket over his red jersey. And the cap was quite a normal one but it had a green stripe in the material.'

'What sort of a man?' I asked.

'Very friendly. Knows everyone in the village and by all accounts quite a scholar.'

'Then he must be Miss Maynard's visitor.'

'I couldn't exactly ask him but I should think very likely.'

It looked as though things were being cleared up at last.

The existence of a real visitor who answered to the description I had been given made all the difference. Miss Maynard was normal and was anxious to protect her maid from outside investigation. Now that I knew this I wanted to see her once more. I hadn't called on her for several weeks and could visit her again without impropriety. I made what amounted to a social call, with the object of letting her know I understood the situation of the household and would not dream of interfering.

'Do you still have visits from your Thursday friend?' I asked after our general chat began to subside.

'Oh he still comes to see me sometimes, but I know who he is now. He is a most interesting man. He reads a lot and we talk about books.'

'Does he still wear his red jersey?'

She looked puzzled for a moment. 'Did I tell you that? Yes he did wear bright clothes at first. I don't notice them now.'

'What about the green striped cap?' I tried to conceal my curiosity by laughing.

'He still wears a cap. You seem very interested in his clothes.'

'You must forgive me. But the first time I saw you you told me you had a strange visitor who came to tea with you every Thursday. You didn't know who he was but he was fat and wore a tight red jersey and a striped green and white cap. I pictured someone like Tweedledum or Tweedledee.'

'Now I begin to see.' She smiled and nodded several times. 'Now I understand. When you first saw me I told you such a strange tale that you wondered whether it was Elsa or me who was telling the truth — who was a little odd in fact. Isn't that right?'

'You are much too clever,' I said.

'Now that we understand each other I will tell you something in strict confidence and then we'll never mention it again. Elsa was in a lot of trouble many years ago and then was kept in care for a long time. I met her when I visited the mental hospital. She was obviously so normal in many ways that I managed to get her out with me on probation. She became devoted to me and has been with me now for ten years or more. I couldn't do without her. And she is a *good* woman. You understand me — a good woman. You once asked me why I had come to live in Somerset. Elsa was one of the reasons. No one knows her past history here.'

'I understand. You have been very good to her.'

'You will know better than I do, but so many people who are called insane are so very nearly normal. Elsa has one very curious tendency — she concerns herself with the people I meet. Sometimes she denies that they exist and sometimes she invents those who don't exist. On our own she is quite normal and so reliable with her work and with money. I would trust her with anything.'

'One last question about her. Why did she telephone me to say you were very ill that day? She said she couldn't wake you up, you remember?'

'Yes. She is terrified that something should happen to me. And it's no wonder, is it? She might have to go back into one of those places. I expect I was asleep, perhaps even snoring a little. Who knows?' Another merry laugh.

That was it, of course. She was asleep and making small noises but with her eyes partly open. Elsa had panicked and rushed to the telephone.

'Thank you for telling me about her. Perhaps I may keep an eye on her? She may come to trust me in time.'

So at last it was all clear to me. The puzzle had been largely of my own making. I had misinterpreted the description of the man who wore an innocent red jersey and imagined a perfectly ordinary cloth cap as having vivid stripes in it. Once the picture of Tweedledum was in my mind I suspected Miss Maynard of hallucinations. Perhaps it was the result of the nettles after all.

I quickly came to love that delightful old lady and saw her from time to time until she died some years later. She carefully left money to provide for Elsa's welfare and the maid survived her by only a few months — a period she spent in a private nursing home.

9

William Pratt suffered from severe pneumokoniosis — dust in the lungs due to work in the collieries. In late middle age his condition was one of the worst I ever encountered. The slow choking as the lungs turned slowly into something as hard and solid as india rubber, the utter inability to expand the chest, the misery of never being able to take a deep breath when the whole body and mind were completely engrossed in an overwhelming desire for air made his life a living hell.

The knowledge that thousands of men, especially in the South Wales and Somerset collieries had died this terrible death made me deeply angry, and having to blame someone, I was angry with colliery owners in general.

I am not sure when the law made this industrial disease a matter for compensation, but when I was first in practice I was told that before a man could claim compensation it was necessary to collect a sample of air from the mine in question, have it analysed and prove it to contain the particles of silica dust that cause the disease. As the disease had been caused by conditions years earlier the absurdity of this process was obvious. By the early nineteen thirties the diagnosis was made entirely by Xray of the lungs. It was easy to demonstrate and compensation then became automatic. By compensation I mean a small pension worth about half the man's normal wages. This would be about a pound a week in the early nineteen thirties, and would of course help towards maintaining a low standard of living. Nothing on earth could compensate for the suffering caused by the disease. If you offered men £100,000 a year to put up with its miseries you would not find a single taker.

103

William Pratt lived and died at a time when the normal compensation of some two pounds a week was paid to him. At least he didn't have to argue or prove in court against all the odds that his health had been ruined by work in the pits. His Xrays proved this clearly enough. All he had to do was to put up with a process of infinitely slow strangulation.

The condition of his lungs slowly caused his heart to fail and this of course added to his distress, but fortunately shortened his suffering by hastening the end. He suffered from this terminal state of affairs for some eighteen months, during which time I was sent for during the night quite frequently — sometimes two or three times a week. The call was always between two and three a.m. when his distress had become intolerable.

What made these night visits different from all others was that instead of cooperation and even a trace of gratitude from his wife, I was faced every time I entered the house by a strangely aggressive posture on her part that was quite remarkable. She behaved as though I was the sole cause of her husband's disability — an attitude that seemed funny at first but became increasingly trying as time went on.

One winter's night I was called out for the third night running to see him. He lived at the end of a row — or rank — of miners' cottages. His bedroom was at the top of the steep stairs and when I arrived he was, as usual, sitting up in bed struggling to breathe. Years ago he had been a powerful man weighing fourteen stone of bone and muscle. Now he had shrunk to little more than half that size. His face was pale grey and moist with sweat in spite of the iciness of the room. His breath was short because his chest could expand, with maximum effort, by a bare half-inch instead of an expansion of about four inches. As he tried to breathe, the muscles of the neck and between the ribs were sucked in by the effort.

He leaned forward, clasping his knees with both hands, living in his own painful separate world where there was only one thought — an intense desire for air. The more he fought the worse he became, because the exertion itself made air even more vitally necessary.

I had seen him like this many times and my reaction was automatic. There was only one possible relief and this was an injection of morphia. I gave him his usual dose and in a few minutes he began to relax and was able to lie back against his high pillows. He would be easy now for a few hours, then the struggle would begin all over again.

As I had left the house on the two previous nights I had been unceremoniously handed a packet of sugar from the little shop run by another member of the Pratt family. It was still the time of rationing and sugar was a luxury, but when it was offered for the third time in three nights it seemed like an automatic payment for my services. The gift was no doubt kindly meant but I felt uncomfortable about it, and that night I protested. The wife was a large woman, not endowed by great sensitivity, and it was difficult to make her understand that I needed no extra payment for a necessary night visit which it was my job to do anyway.

'I can't take any more sugar, Mrs Pratt,' I said. 'You've already given me two packets this week.'

She weighed the sugar in her hand as though striking a bargain. 'I haven't got much butter. I could squeeze half a pound if that's what you der want.'

'I didn't mean that. It's very kind of you but I don't need either. Your husband is a panel patient and you've every right to send for me when he is as bad as this. I'm only doing my job and I don't want to rob anyone else of their rations.'

'I shouldn't be giving un to yer if you was robbin' anyone.'

'Well you keep it. Your husband will be easier now and I'll call and see him again later in the day.'

'Please yerself,' she said with a shrug or a sniff — possibly both.

Evidently I had offended her. Perhaps she felt better for 'paying me' something extra, or under less of an obligation. At that hour in the morning I didn't feel much like arguing or being especially tactful. I only felt that taking the sugar seemed like taking a bribe for doing what I had to do anyway. Perhaps I enjoyed the feeling of martyrdom, of putting people into my debt, I don't know. And yet I hated those frequent night visits.

Then why object to the sugar which they had plenty of and wanted to give me? Was it because the sum of sixty pence a year, which the government paid us for looking after each panel patient, was supposed to cover all treatment including a night visit every night of the year if necessary? Was I that conscientious? Or was it Mrs Pratt's manner? That was nearer the truth. I didn't like to feel beholden to an aggressive woman.

I often wondered what made her so aggressive and how I should respond. Once, years before, I had had a lesson on the treatment of aggression and had it in mind to put this to the test. I had been walking with an uncle of mine in the country when an apparently mad dog flew at us with ears back and teeth bared. My reaction was to fight him off with my stick which had a point at the end, but my uncle stood quite still and said quietly, 'I wonder what's troubling him. He's badly upset by something.'

We stood still for a full minute watching the dog slowly settle down. At last he became quiet and looked at us questioningly, then turned round and slunk off. My uncle said 'alright old friend, we're quite harmless' or words to that effect and the dog turned for a second and looked at us again before making off altogether. If I had defended myself with my pointed stick we should have been facing the animal for hours.

When I thought of that ferocious dog I began to ask myself whether it would be possible to deal with an aggressive human being in the same way. This I found extremely difficult because my own aggressions became fierce as soon as I was — or even imagined I was — being attacked. Even now I have not completely learned the lesson, but with Mrs Pratt I tried to take the first step.

In time I learned what I thought was the cause of her antagonism. She was disturbed every night and had to work hard all day. She had a son and a daughter living at home and going out to work. It is imperative to some people to have at hand someone to blame when things go wrong, and she was one of these. Things had not only gone

106

badly wrong for her but she must have felt perpetually exhausted.

In the early hours of one morning she said bitterly, 'No one do know what he do suffer and all he do get is a few shillin' compensation. If one of *them* 'ad to put up wi' what 'e does they'd be screaming murder.'

'They didn't know how to prevent it when Will got his trouble,' I replied. 'Nowadays they do a lot more to keep the dust down, especially after the shot-firing. They won't let the men go back where they've used an explosive till the dust is well settled.'

'You'd take their part of course.' The sarcasm was heavy.

'I'm not taking anyone's part,' I said hotly. 'This dust disease is one of the worst things that can happen to a man. But once he's got it all we can do is to ease him as best we can. The only thing is to prevent it from happening and that's what they are trying to do.'

'What good's that going to do Will?'

'None, I'm afraid.'

'Then why do 'e take their part?'

I was torn between sympathy for poor Will's suffering and my reaction to the wife's habit of seeming to blame me for all his troubles. It was bad enough to be called out every other night, but worse still to go into the lion's den where every agonised breath was firmly put down to my supposedly being in league with the employers.

'You always say 'tis the men's own fault for not keeping out the way long enough after the shot-firin'. But that ain't true. Will always obeyed the rules. But years ago they was told to get on and bring the coal out.'

'Shot-firing wasn't all of it, of course,' I said. 'When they drilled through the rock when they were sinking the shafts some of that graze was very hard. A lot of men got their dust disease while they were drilling.'

'Twasn't the men's fault whatever you do say.'

No matter how conciliatory I tried to be or how I explained the causes of the disease my words were twisted to suggest that I thought it was always due to the men's carelessness. I was identified with the enemy, the employers,

107

the unseen ones who had caused her husband's disease. Unfair, of course, but that is how many people's minds work. The fact was, I kept telling myself, that the poor woman was at her wits' end with fatigue and had to lash out at someone. I felt sure that if she could meet some of the employers face to face she might realise that they were nearly as distressed by the disease as she was.

No one at that time had thought of trying to make euthanasia legal and the thought of giving him an over-dose of morphia never entered my head. Looking back there was much to be said for shortening his life. He was incapable of any sort of normal living, even for a few minutes. His struggle to breathe was constant and his brain was suffering from a continual lack of oxygen, making his state of mind one long nightmare. Morphia, of course, gave only temporary relief and as its effects wore off his distress was as great or greater than ever. Nowadays it is likely that such cases would be admitted to one of the splendid hospices for the incurable, where relief would be given constantly whatever its effect on the length of life.

One day I met one of the colliery owners. Alcohol was becoming somewhat more easily available and we met at one of the first Sunday morning drinks parties after the war. Jessica and I arrived late and there was the usual noise of raised voices. My instinct was to turn and run but I was led firmly into the noise and heat of battle. On those occasions I have often thought of the words of W.H. Auden's poem — The Party — where he describes the vigorous conversation in which everyone talks and no one listens, where they look constantly over their shoulders to see if there is someone else more interesting to talk to, where they utter a 'howl for recognition fraught with fear'. Will no one listen to me? I saw John Bossingham across the room and made my way over to him. He was one of the younger and more active owners, and I broached the subject of pneumokoniosis and William Pratt. I asked him whether conditions in the pits had improved enough to prevent further cases of this horrible disease.

'You'll never prevent it altogether,' he said, or rather shouted so that I could just hear him. 'A lot of it's the men's own fault. They won't do as they're told.'

He was going to trot out the old argument about the men not waiting for the dust to clear after using explosives. This reminded me of the suggestion that council houses should not have bathrooms because the tenants would only keep their coal in the bath, so I forestalled him.

'You mean after the explosive is put in deep-drilled holes and fired, the men won't keep away till the dust is cleared. I understand that, but even after that the dust is only on the ground. It must come up into the air again whenever they work in the area. Isn't there some method of properly ventilating the pits so that the dust can be carried away altogether?'

'There are ways of course, but they are expensive. You'd have to sink shafts all over the place and blow air through at regular intervals. No one could afford that. Most of the dust can be settled by water on the ground and water on the rock while they are drilling, of course. We've been doing that for years.'

'Have you ever seen a man suffering from the advanced stages of pneumokoniosis?'

'I can't say I've seen them at their worst but I know it's a rotten thing to have.'

'Would you like to come and see one of your men in the late stages?'

This was a challenge and he hesitated, then began to fumble with his diary saying that he was very busy. 'Would it serve any useful purpose?' he asked.

'I think it might influence your ideas about preventive measures,' I said, 'however expensive they are.'

'The government will be taking over soon so it hardly concerns us now.'

'Will they be prepared to spend what is necessary to control the dust?'

'I suppose so.'

'It may not be for some time. Will you come and see this man?'

'What good will it do?'

'It will increase your understanding of what dust disease is really like.'

'I do understand it, I assure you. Anyway it's a bit too late in the day now I'm afraid.'

'There's the question of compensation too.'

At this word his attitude hardened. I had seen both sides of the problem and understood how he felt about it. I had seen men claiming compensation they had no earthly right to, and others paid a mere pittance for the complete ruin of their health. The thought occurred to me that by taking Mr Bossingham to see Pratt I might make him look at industrial relations from another angle.

'If the man you're talking about has genuine pneumo-koniosis he will be receiving compensation.'

'Yes, two pounds a week.'

'That is decided by the law of the land. It's not our affair.'

'I know that but I would like you to come and see him.'

Bossingham was essentially a decent man. He and his colleagues had been forced to struggle desperately in the past to make the pits pay their way. Because of the sins of their predecessors in a very different world they had inherited an unjustified reputation for ruthlessness. Suddenly he made up his mind.

'Alright, I'll see him. Bring him to the manager's office at the colliery — say. . . .' He looked again at his diary but I interrupted him.

'He's much too ill for that,' I said.

He looked at me in surprise. 'You mean you want me to come to his house? How would that be interpreted by the union?'

'As a sign of personal interest in your employees, of course.'

'Alright. Let's go and see him now.'

'Right.' We were both rather glad to escape the noise and there and then we made our excuses to our host. I arranged for Jessica to have a lift home with a neighbour and in five minutes I was knocking at the door of the Pratts' cottage.

I led the way up the steep stairs to the bedroom where

Pratt was sitting up in bed as usual. There was one small window in the room, facing over a tiny garden and giving a view of nothing but some bare cabbage stumps and beyond that the rising ground that led to the colliery. It was a vivid contrast to the room and garden we had just left.

The bedroom contained, besides an iron bedstead, a washstand with bowl and jug, two wooden chairs and a chamber-pot half hidden under the bed. There was, too, a large wooden box probably used for storing and as an extra seat or surface. Some clothes were hanging neatly against one wall and the place was scrupulously clean. I was momentarily conscious of being relieved that we had not embarrassed Mrs Pratt by catching her unawares.

'I've brought Mr Bossingham to see you, Pratt,' I said. 'He is concerned at the amount of trouble you are getting with your breathing.'

Pratt raised a hand automatically and said 'Good morning sir'. His colour was pale grey and his breathing restricted as usual. With loss of weight the skin now lay in folds round his neck.

Mr Bossingham said he was sorry to hear that Pratt had been so ill and then seemed at a loss. He had none of the skills of those lay men or women who visit the sick regularly. He walked to the window and stood with his back to it, looking at the patient.

I asked Pratt a few questions about where he had worked in the pit and how long — questions I knew the answer to, but which seemed to be what the visitor should be asking. Then I loosened his nightshirt so as to expose his chest. 'Just show us how difficult your breathing is,' I said. 'Take a deep breath.'

The chest expanded by its usual half an inch. There was little cough as a rule but it so happened that day that he had some catarrh which was worrying him. He began to cough violently and this with his restricted chest movement made him almost lose consciousness. He fought for breath for several minutes while we stood impotently by. The sight was pitiful to look at but I was glad in one way that his true plight could be seen so quickly.

We watched the short shallow breathing for several minutes while he slowly regained his stability. I could feel the tension and embarrassment mounting in my guest, and when I felt sure the man's misery was well and truly noted I told Pratt I would see him again tomorrow and led the way downstairs.

I wondered whether Mrs Pratt would show her temper to the visitor, but she was overcome by his presence and kept silence. Bossingham managed to say he was very sorry for Pratt's trouble and would do all he could to help. Then with obvious relief he accompanied me back to the car. Once there he took out a cigarette, lighted it and inhaled deeply. 'Poor bastard,' he said. Then he became defensive. 'I don't feel any responsibility myself. He developed that in my predecessor's time. We're doing our best to keep the air clean now.'

He was silent on our way back to where we had left his car and I thought there was nothing to be gained by talking about the case. Pratt had done everything possible to show what pneumokoniosis meant. Before he left me Bossingham commented, 'I've always said that nationalisation is the only thing for the mines. They need a fortune spent on them to prevent what that poor devil's got.'

I wondered later whether I had done any good to industrial relations by pressing him to make the call. Probably none whatever. I had however done myself good. I no longer felt a deep vague sense of grievance against colliery owners.

When I called on the Pratts next day Mrs Pratt was as aggressive as ever. 'What did er want to come pryin' here for?' she said.

'The only way we can get conditions in the pits improved,' I told her, 'is by letting the owners know what really happens to the men who get dust disease.'

'So it was your doin'? You did tell un to come?'

'I did, yes.'

'And how much good did that do to my Will?'

'None, Mrs Pratt. None. I know that.'

That morning Pratt was clear-headed and this meant that he was slightly stronger but in greater suffering. To be fully aware of the pain and strain and to know that it would only be relieved by death was a grim state. When his mind began to wander or he was in an uneasy dream he probably suffered less. That day was one of his worst.

'I ain't goin' to no 'ospital.' His voice was weak and every word he spoke had to be essential to make the effort worth while. He had evidently been thinking that the colliery owner would want him moved to hospital if anything was to be done to help. This was useless and I told him there was no question to it.

In hospital he would be given oxygen which would afford temporary relief but would prolong his life and misery. Morphia in sufficient quantities to give real relief was the only humane treatment. Not being a surgical case he was not eligible for a bed in the cottage hospital and, even if they had given him a bed in the city hospital, he was better off at home.

I visited him several times a day towards the end and still had to defend myself against Mrs Pratt. 'Can't 'e do summat to ease 'im?' she asked time after time, to which I would reply, 'There's nothing more anyone could do for him. The morphia is the only thing.'

Then at last she demanded a specialist. 'We'll pay for someone to come out from Bath,' she said. 'If you can't do no more than this we must 'ave someone.'

I welcomed the idea of sharing the responsibility though I knew no one could help. The trouble was that the Pratts could not possibly afford the fee of ten guineas, and such a sacrifice for no benefit made me hesitate.

'You bain't doin un no good at all and perhaps there's summat you don't know about.' I still hesitated and perhaps she read my thoughts. 'You get the specialist. We'll pay for un.'

When I explained the case to one of the Bath physicians he offered to come out without charging a fee at all. He did so, and confirmed that no more could be done for poor Pratt. He backed my treatment, paying the usual supporting compliment that helped us with our patients. After this I expected Mrs Pratt to be more friendly or at least less aggressive, but she didn't change.

113

'If we 'ad more money 'e wouldn't say that,' she said. 'Tis one thing ver the rich and another ver the poor as usual.'

Every day I told myself that her manner was nothing to do with me personally, and that she was under such severe strain that it was good for her to have someone to blame. I began to pride myself on my patience with her.

Pratt died at last. The post-mortem showed the expected india rubber lungs and the official compensation was paid to the widow. His was a sad story and I hoped desperately that under nationalisation more would be done to prevent the disease. More was done, of course, and the increase in the cost of coal was a small price to pay for the better conditions.

Sometimes after you have spent a great deal of time in attendance on a dying patient, one of the relatives will write a letter of thanks. Sometimes one of them will come and thank you personally and this gives you a feeling of satisfaction at having done your best. I felt I had been very attentive and very patient and understanding with Mrs Pratt. I was, in fact, rather pleased with myself and firmly expected some mark of appreciation. None came, but at last I had a letter from one of Pratt's sons. I opened it with the thought that it was better late than never.

The letter stated briefly that the whole family intended to transfer to Dr Braythwaite. There was no complaint, no thanks, just a plain statement of fact. I was flabbergasted. Never had I given more unstinted attention to a patient by day and by night. Never had I done so many night visits for one patient. Why, I wondered, had they taken offence. Years later some of the younger members of the family came back to me but I never saw Mrs Pratt again.

It was, I suppose, a simple matter of 'I do not like you Dr Fell, the reason why I cannot tell'. Looking back, I believe it would have been wiser to have given her a piece of my mind instead of trying so hard to understand her, constantly making allowances for her. Patience and understanding are often less effective than natural behaviour. She needed someone to stand up to her, so no doubt Will had done in the past. If there is a rule for human conduct it is 'be yourself, be natural.'

The transfer to the new National Health Service was only

a few months ahead and I began to wonder how I should face. It was impossible at that time to know how many patients one had. We knew the number of panel patients we were responsible for, but you never knew whether a family had kept in good health for a long time or whether they had transferred to another doctor. The delightful old world courtesy of prewar days, when every doctor would telephone his colleague if a patient transferred to him, had gone for ever.

I seemed always busy but that wasn't much to go by. I had about eleven hundred panel patients which ought to indicate that I should have some two thousand seven hundred patients altogether, but I had many doubts and schooled myself to be prepared for humiliation. If the Pratts wanted to transfer to the opposition after all I had done for them, many others might do the same. For the first time everyone was to be given a card to take to the doctor of their choice and the choice was absolutely free. They need have no allegiance to anyone, and all those who had long wanted to transfer to another doctor but hadn't liked to do so could at last go where they pleased.

In a few months we should know what our patients really thought of us, and after the Pratt affair I was not at all sure!

10

Beth, our youngest daughter who was six at the time, would have told you that there were eight people living in our house — mother, father, four children, one maid and 'the-telephone'. The-telephone was an abrasive disturbing character who had to be continually supervised, like a demanding crippled patient who must never be left alone. 'Who's going to look after the telephone?' someone would ask if we were thinking of going out. It was very much alive, the one discordant member of the household, the black sheep of the family.

It would scream at you as you came through the door at the end of a tiring day, or as you put the first mouthful of your meal on the fork, or when you slid into bed at night, or worst of all when you were in that deep essential sleep of the early morning hours that renewed your sanity and revitalised all the organs of your body.

I remember Beth coming down the stairs one morning while I was drinking my coffee at breakfast. 'The telephone hasn't gone all the morning,' she said as though it was already nearly lunch-time.

'Careful,' I whispered, 'or you'll make it go.' Poor child, no wonder she thought it was alive. And of course at that precise moment it rang.

It was old Lyddy Barlow, the maid who had looked after Eustace Broddick since his second wife had died a year earlier. 'It's the master,' she shouted. 'He's in agony. He can't move nor hand nor foot. I think it might be a stroke.'

'Where is the pain?' I asked her.

'His back and his stomach mostly,' then for good measure, 'and his legs and his shoulders.'

116

I waited for her to add that his chest and his head were also affected but she had already rung off. Obviously she was in a panic and equally clearly Eustace Broddick was in serious pain. It didn't sound like a stroke but the pain might have been anything from gall-stones to a heart attack, and it meant an urgent visit. It was fortunate that I knew where he lived because Lyddy hadn't mentioned an address.

I swallowed the rest of my coffee, kissed my youngest daughter who was looking as though she was entirely responsible for the emergency, and set out for Rapton where Mr Broddick lived. We still had no appointment system at that time and I was due in the surgery in ten minutes. To start at the offical hour of nine o'clock meant a day of never catching up with the work. I always did my best to be in my consulting-room by half-past eight but today old Eustace — it was inevitable that I should refer to him in my own mind as 'Useless' — was going to take up the vital half-hour of the morning that was bound to ruin my day.

It was a fine morning and the July sunshine did something to raise my spirits. I knew I had a full day ahead and if Eustace had gall-stone or renal colic — the two major pains in everyday experience — he might need several visits before bedtime. Pain relief and some hours of observation would certainly precede any possible admission to hospital.

He was an interesting character. He had held a senior position in local government in a Midland town before he retired and came to live in Rapton. He was seventy-one years old, slim, well preserved, his hair thin but thanks to artificial aid still dark. He had charming manners, made you feel quickly at home and listened carefully to everything you said. On the other hand he was a rigid character, well satisfied with his own opinions and apt to attribute any difference with another person to their ignorance or error or both. 'In matters controversial, my perception's very fine, I always see two points of view, the one that's wrong and mine,' might have been his favourite verse but he would have used the words seriously, with no hint of poking fun at himself.

He must have had something of a private fortune because he lived very comfortably in a good-sized house with two resident maids, when most people of the middle classes had none or at the most one. He was a good bridge-player, reputedly quite an expert at chess, and spent much of his time at one or other of the games.

I found him in acute pain but suffering from nothing more serious than lumbago, as we called it then before prolapsed disks became the most frequently diagnosed condition of the day. His lumbar muscles were in violent spasm and movement was virtually impossible. I gave him pain relief, arranged for his mattress to be supported by a board and promised to call on him the next day.

My reason for recording this seemingly routine visit is that it had a profound effect on several lives. He took the usual time to settle down and after a fortnight he told me the reason for his impatience to get better. He was going to be married again.

My first reaction was one of pleasure. He had been very lonely since his wife died and no doubt his health and wellbeing, as well as his spirits, would improve with the benefit of companionship.

'I think you know my fiancée,' he said. 'She is a patient of yours, I understand. Her name is Marjorie Fallows.'

I was startled and must have failed completely to disguise my feelings. Marjorie was an attractive young woman whom I had known since she was a child. She was a miner's daughter who now worked in a fashion shop in the city. She was twenty-five. I found myself wondering how on earth he could have met her.

I managed to congratulate him on his good fortune but couldn't bring myself to say anything more. Perhaps my tone annoyed him and he spoke with some asperity. 'I suppose you think she is too young or that I am too old.'

'There's a lot of difference between your ages but I hope you will be very happy.'

'Perhaps you understand now why I am somewhat bothered about this back trouble. I don't want Marjorie to get the impression that she is marrying a cripple.'

'No one would think that. You are very fit for your age and of course this lumbago can affect people at any time of life.'

'I'm glad you say that. I'm very lucky, I know. She's a very beautiful girl.'

Marjorie was certainly not beautiful. She was attractive because she was young, vivacious and healthy.

You might say it was no business of mine but in general practice the affairs of your patients are your business. Their health depends on their way of life and their relationships — especially their marriages. Not that I would suggest that we should see our patients as potential clients at a marriage bureau, or try to influence personal decisions of that sort, but we had a right to be concerned.

In 1947, 'affairs' — meaning bouts of adultery — were very rare in the country, and marriage was regarded as a matter of permanence. I confess to having felt mildly distressed to hear that a young, healthy and attractive girl was proposing to tie herself to a man of seventy-one — old enough to be not only her father but her grandfather. If Marjorie Fallows had been a psychological case or a lesbian it would not have been so bad, but she was neither of these. I knew she had been engaged to a young man and the engagement had fallen through not long ago, and I knew that her father had been killed in a pit accident when she was a child. It was possible that she was mentally marrying a father figure because the loss of her father at an impressionable age had had traumatic effects, but I couldn't hope to understand fully why she should marry a man of Broddick's age.

Since that time I have known marriages with equal age differences which turned out to be highly successful, but at that time I had less experience and found the affair rather depressing.

The worst aspect of all was that I knew that both Eustace Broddick's marriages had run into difficulties. His first wife, whom I had not known, had apparently become a severe neurotic and the marriage had ended in divorce. His second wife had seemed a strong-minded woman during the short time I had known her. She had died suddenly of a heart attack. But he had once told me in confidence that both his marriages had been 'a mistake', and I began to wonder whether Marjorie Fallows was destined to become the third 'mistake'.

'You told me once,' I said, 'that both your marriages were — mistakes was the word you used. What did you mean exactly? I didn't know the first Mrs Broddick but I knew your second wife. I had no idea you had had serious trouble then.'

He looked at me appraisingly for a moment. 'I suppose you are the right person to discuss the matter with. I don't know who else I can talk to.' I waited while he made up his mind. At last he went on, 'I think I'm a healthy man in every way but both my wives were — you can only call it oversexed. We were not well matched. That is why I said both marriages were a mistake. A matter of luck I suppose, that sort of thing.'

'I think it's a good plan to talk about it, as you are marrying again.'

'It's difficult to talk about, but that is the only way I can express it.'

'Did you ever get advice about it?'

'Advice? What could that do? You couldn't change the nature of either of them. I was very fond of them but — that was the case.'

'The question is why you found them both incompatible. As it happened with two separate women it makes one wonder.'

'I don't find anything to wonder about. They were both oversexed. Now Marjorie — she's different.'

'You mean she doesn't seem so interested in sex?'

'It's not so simple as that. I think she is a very normal young woman but she doesn't over-emphasise that element of life.'

'It's always a problem to know that until you are married,' I said. He was a sensitive man, and I felt doubts about the effect of telling him there was probably much about sex that he didn't understand.

'I don't think we shall have any problems, Doctor.' He spoke dismissively and it was impossible to pursue the matter further.

My concern was that most so-called oversexed women suffered in fact from ineffective husbands. It would be sad to think of Majorie Fallows sacrificing herself not only to an old man, but to a man who rather arrogantly blamed two women for being oversexed when they had probably been victims of his own abnormality or ignorance.

There was always the problem in those days of getting people to talk freely on this subject. Marie Stopes had written wisely many years ago and Van de Welde had written wisely, scientifically and copiously on the subject, but whereas in the nineteen eighties sex is an easy topic of conversation, in the nineteen forties it was still taboo to the majority of people. I should get nowhere with Eustace Broddick and should have to leave the matter alone. My guess was that he was either too ignorant or too selfish to make a good husband, although it was possible that he suffered some degree of abnormality. Today it would be easy to ask point blank questions, but in those days it would have been unthinkable. Most people would shut up like a clam as soon as their personal sex lives were questioned. Not for the first time my sympathies went out to Marie Stopes, who had fought a long lone battle on behalf of thousands of misunderstood women only to become the subject of bawdy jokes. She was a pioneer but 'rich in saving common sense'.

My only hope was that Marjorie Fallows would consult me before her marriage and this was unlikely in those days. If by chance she did I might be able to talk to her about possible problems. Even so she would have to be a remarkably strong-minded young woman to be able to undertake the education of Eustace Broddick.

I heard that the wedding was due to take place fairly shortly — I think it was in September that year. My own opinions were unorthodox at that time and I had expressed them freely. I believe now and believed then that any couple who intended marriage should live together beforehand for a time, to be sure there were no insuperable sex problems. I think this practice should be preceded by the formality of betrothal, so as to eliminate as far as possible the habit of using it as an excuse for promiscuity. Once married I believed that the union should be permanent except in cases of extreme difficulty. My opinions were of course frowned on by orthodox churchmen but I was heartened to find a very understanding attitude from others. It was some years later that I expressed my opinions in an article in the medical periodical *Pulse* and on the day of publication the BBC contacted me before ten in the morning to ask for an interview. This was recorded amicably until the last question nearly floored me. 'What do you tell your own daughters to do?' Fortunately I was able to say they were all married by then and so escaped an answer that might have embarrassed them!

Marjorie did not consult me on the subject of her marriage. She did however have an accident. She fell and broke her wrist. The frequency with which so-called accidents interfere with dramatic force in the course of life has always struck me. I think years later Dr Michael Balint would have attributed this to the 'emotional component' in the causation of accidents. He would say that many accidents are not a matter of chance, that they sometimes occur as a result of a suppressed element of will on the part of the patient. Certainly they happen more frequently during periods of strain and sometimes help in the solution of problems.

I had Marjorie Xrayed, corrected the displacement in her wrist and put her in plaster of Paris. Naturally there was no opportunity to talk of her marriage at first, but I did ask later if it would have to be postponed.

'I don't want it to be but I shan't make a very good wife like this.'

It was clear that I should do no good unless I took the plunge and asked a direct question. 'Marjorie,' I said, 'I have known you since you were a small girl. Are you perfectly happly about marrying someone as old as Mr Broddick?'

'Yes, perfectly happy,' she said. And that was that.

'You were engaged, weren't you, till a few months ago to a young man?'

'A very young man, yes. He was three years younger than me.'

'Don't answer if you don't want to, but have you any experience of sex?'

She blushed and said, 'I have in a way.'

'And are you sure you can be happy with a much older man?'

'Marriage is not only about sex.'

'True, but sex is a big part of it. Has Mr Broddick talked to you about his earlier marriages?'

'Yes. I think — he was rather unlucky.'

'Did he tell you that he thought both his marriages were a mistake?'

'He said both his wives were — sort of oversexed.'

'Well, that means that the relationship between him and both his wives was unsatisfactory. Does it strike you that it might not have been the wives who were the cause of the trouble?'

Her face became crimson as she began to see what I was driving at. 'I don't quite understand what you mean,' she said.

'Quite often when a woman is said to be oversexed it's the man's fault, and she's not oversexed at all. Have you read any books about it?'

'No.'

'Then I think you should.' I wrote down the names of two books I recommended. 'If Mr Broddick had one wife he thought oversexed that wouldn't be very remarkable, but as he has had two I think you should consider the possibility that he was responsible for their unsatisfactory lives.' All the time one had to skate round direct statements which would have made everything so much clearer, but which would have driven the patient away behind a wall of embarrassment and ended all hope of real understanding.

'You mean he is not very strong in that way?'

'Not necessarily. There are a number of causes of breakdown of that side of marriage. To begin with, men and women have different approaches. Most men are ready for sex at any time. Women are obviously not. They need to be wooed, if you like the word. If the man doesn't take care over this the woman may feel worse than if she had no husband at all. Do you understand what I'm trying to say? There are some things that you can only find out when you live with each other.'

She was silent and thoughtful. 'I think I understand'.

Advice like this, which sounds so elementary in the nineteen eighties, was very necessary in the forties. Reluctantly now she rose to go. I couldn't say any more unless she asked for help. I wondered whether I had been wise or foolish. On one previous occasion when I had spoken to a couple in this way I had been greeted by a stony silence, and much later found that they had long been perfectly adapted to each other. Anyway I had tried to help this girl, and if she took no notice of what I said there was nothing more I could do.

Next time I saw her she told me that the wedding had been postponed for a month. This would do nothing but good in any case.

I saw Eustace Broddick at about the same time. His back had recovered and I told him to avoid lifting in awkward positions and sitting too long in deep armchairs. He listened carefully as usual, then referred to the postponement of his marriage.

'Marjorie was very unfortunate. She tripped down those steps and I feel sure some hooligan had thrown some rubbish on them. She would never have fallen otherwise. She comes down them every day. So now I have to wait another month before I can bring her home here.'

I wanted to say 'Why wait? Why not learn more about each other before you commit yourselves?' I imagined his reaction to such an outrageous suggestion. He would probably have walked quietly to the door, opened it for me and said, 'I will let you know if I require your services again.' My thoughts must have caused a ghost of a smile because I was puzzled for a moment by what he said next.

'You find the prospect amusing?'

'Not in the least,' I said. 'I sympathise with you but she should be quite recoverd by the end of a month — except for a stiff wrist for a time.'

Some mild antagonism seemed to have developed between us, whereas previously we had been good friends. Thoughts are powerful things and I must confess I was distressed by what I regarded as this unsuitable marriage.

I saw Marjorie, probably to give her a panel certificate.

She was still in plaster. 'I read one of those books,' she said.

'Did you find it helpful?'

'Not really. It seemed to make a lot of complications over something that is after all quite natural.'

Once more I found the woman in the case far more easy to talk to than the man. 'Quite natural, yes, but you only have to look at all the unhappy marriages there are around to know that what is natural is not always simple. Monogamy and marriage are neither so natural or so simple as they might be. Perhaps cavemen had easy solutions to their problems, but modern men and women often find difficulties. Knowledge is better than ignorance in the long run.'

'I wondered whether Eustace would read the book so I took it to him.'

'How did he react?'

'Not very well. He said all this scientific analysis only turned something very beautiful into an exercise in biology.'

'Did that convince you?'

'No. I'm not very confident about the future. Sometimes I wish I could talk to him more freely.'

'A lot of men are very reluctant to talk about these things. But you're a woman. You have enormous power in your hands — at present.'

I hoped the last two words would sink in and she looked at me as though wondering what to say next. I handed her a certificate and waited. She folded it and put it in her handbag, taking time in the simple operation because of her plastered arm. Then she said 'Thank you for trying to help.'

I wanted to say, 'Go and sleep with him. Get to know more about him.' But I knew it wouldn't do.

I didn't see her for a fortnight and then I was confronted by a completely changed woman. She was self-assured and frank as women often are on this subject when they set their minds to it.

'I decided there was only one way to find out whether Eustace and I would be happy together. I spent several nights with him. I expect this shocks you.'

'Not in the least,' I said. 'To be honest that's what I hoped you would do, although I couldn't very well suggest it myself. You were very wise. Now is the time to find out whether you are suited to each other or not.' I waited.

'We decided to put the wedding off for a while. He suggested it, not me, but we both agreed about it.'

'I'm glad you are taking time. It's a very important decision.' I would like to have known what had happened during those nights but had no right to ask.

'You know he's got no children. He wants one very much. I think perhaps he wants a child more than he wants me.'

And with these gentle hints as to what had happened between them I had to be satisfied.

I had completed my treatment of Eustace Broddick's lumbago but wanted very much to see him again. One day when I was passing through Rapton I stopped at his house. He was at home and I asked about his back and his general health. Marjorie Fallows might or might not have mentioned my name to him. If she had I might have been blamed for interference, but apparently she hadn't.

Presently I brought up the subject of his marriage. 'I understand you have postponed the wedding for a time,' I said.

He seemed to consider and then decided to become confidential. 'I've been having second thoughts,' he told me.

'Have you?' I waited.

'Perhaps she is too young after all.'

'You and she are the only ones who can decide that.'

'To be quite honest, Doctor — you know I've never talked about these matters before to a living soul — I'm wondering whether I'm such a good husband after all.'

'It's all a matter of compatibility, isn't it? Sexual compatibility in fact. People vary so much and the only way to be sure that a couple are well matched is by marriage or a trial marriage.'

'Are you suggesting that people should live together before they are married?'

'Yes.'

'Don't you regard that as immoral?'

126

'No. I regard it as a sensible precaution. The greatest disaster is for a marriage to break down, especially when there are children. It is worth a great deal to prevent that.'

'I wonder whether it would prevent it.'

'It would rule out one major cause of breakdown.'

'And what would our clergy friends say about it?'

'Eventually I think they will have to accept it — at least not to condemn those who take that precaution.'

'What happens if the woman becomes pregnant and then decides she has got the wrong man?'

'She would never let that happen. There are plenty of birth control clinics if they don't know what to do about it.'

Broddick became thoughtful and I guessed he was asking himself what Marjorie Fallows had done about this particular problem. I was sure he didn't know about her talks with me.

Months went by and the two were not married. Finally I heard that the engagement had been broken off. I was pleased and the case soon drifted into the enlarging limbo in my mind of half-forgotten histories.

Marjorie Fallows was married to a man of her own age within a year or so and it was when I attended her in her first confinement that I heard the end of the story. I often think how much family doctors miss by not attending their patients' confinements. You learn more about the men and women under your care in a few hours at those times than in years of routine.

'I've got a lot to thank you for,' she said. I was visiting her one evening and she sat placidly feeding her baby. 'You helped me make up my mind about that other engagement.'

'How did I do that?' I asked.

'You told me he had probably been a bad husband to two wives already, you remember?'

'I remember. He said they had both been mistakes.'

'Well I should have been his third mistake if it hadn't been for you.'

'I never understood how a girl like you could fall in love with a man fifty years older than yourself.'

127

'It's hard to explain. But I was very fond of him. It was soon after I broke off my first engagement. And he was very charming, so kind and thoughtful. He did so want a child and I still feel sorry for him.'

'But you bravely found out more about him. I remember. Do you want to talk about it?'

'I'd rather forget it. But you were quite right. I shudder to think what might have happened.'

'You are happy enough now?'

'Yes, very happy. We fight sometimes but we love as well.'

'It takes a young man to do both properly.'

Eustace Broddick never married again. He lived ten years of apparently contented old age. Sometimes I wondered whether my influence on Marjorie Fallows had robbed him of a lot of happiness, but on the whole my conscience was easy.

My opinion about trial marriages has not changed. Years after the episode related here I talked to a close old friend Edward Tyndall who always gave me the benefit of frank criticism.

'Your idea of trial marriages hasn't done much good,' he said. 'The divorce rate is getting worse every year.'

'I know it is, but it's not the result of trial marriages. It's due to the acceptance of adultery as part of the natural order of things.'

He shrugged in a characteristic way he had.

'The stability of marriage depends on the sex bond,' I went on. 'If your only sexual partner is your husband or your wife you'll tend to stick together through thick and thin. With promiscuity you break the main bond. Hence the frequent divorces and the psychological damage to children.'

'For once,' he said, 'for once you might be more right than usual.' And I was convinced I was.

11

Every year in May we had a holiday together, the two of us. They were holidays we couldn't really afford because school fees soon dominated our budget. At the same time we knew that those happy years would never come again. We were permanently in love, apart from those occasional bursts of mutual fury that serve only to heighten the joys of normal times, and after these brief storms our separate selves would come together again with the completeness of a chemical fusion.

The difference between us was often highlighted on holiday when Jessica would become entranced in one of the great art galleries. Perhaps it would be a painting by Andrea del Sarto. One day she sat spellbound in Munich for over half an hour looking at an Assumption of the Madonna by Guido Reni. I enjoyed her pleasure but couldn't share it. I soon came to know that the work of the world's great artists was not for my enjoyment or inspiration. We visited in the course of the years all the great galleries of Europe except the Hermitage in Leningrad. In time I began to get some degree of pleasure from the colours and forms and especially the characters revealed in the faces the artists left for us. Ghirlandaio's old man with cysts on his nose and the trusting child for instance, Leonardo's face of St Martha in The Virgin of the Rocks and Michelangelo's Adam all impressed me enough to make me hang copies of them in my room.

By no means all our holidays were centred on the galleries. There were breakfasts on the balconies of Swiss hotels, picnics consisting of French cheeses, rolls and a bottle of wine, explorations of the countryside, visits to the opera in Vienna, and all these things gave equal pleasure to both of us.

In May 1947 we had our first foreign holiday after the war. We were allowed only £25 each to spend out of England but they were splendid, solid and respected pounds. This amount was just within our budget limits and that year we managed nine days in a Swiss village. It was our first visit to Switzerland, magical and romantic. We were welcomed particularly warmly because we were British — almost as though we were personally responsible for winning the war. There were few English tourists and none with money to spare, yet the skilful Swiss hoteliers made us feel and live like princes. They fed us as though we were children who had been starved for the six years of war. We climbed mountains, picked gentians (only a very few!) looked with reverence at soldenella, trolleus, alpine roses, sulphur flowers and the occasional eidelweiss, sat in carriages drawn by horses bedecked with flowers that took us on day trips to local beauty spots. We basked in the sunshine and blue skies that fittingly celebrated the coming of peace to shattered Europe. We were both just over forty — surely the finest time of human life!

When we left our village and boarded the spotlessly clean Swiss train, passed through stations decorated with flowers and left the mountains behind, Jessica's tears flowed freely and my own expression must have been that of one who sadly looks on at the end of the world. Nothing, we thought, could ever match that holiday. Yet others did, time after time. We came to be glad that we had at least suffered some hardship and separation during the war. Else life would have been too good.

Directly after our holiday that year the great debate on the coming of the National Health Service got into full swing. The majority of doctors were vehemently opposed to taking any part in it. We should lose our freedom, they said, we should be dragooned, bullied and regimented, told how we must treat our patients, forced to prescribe only second-class drugs, the age-old relationship between doctor and patient would be lost for ever — and so on and so on.

I was strongly in favour of some sort of health service financed by national insurance. The childhood experience of watching my father financially crippled by the three years of my mother's illness before she died was deeply ingrained in my thinking. Every assistance to health like good medical treatment, clean air and pure water was everyone's birthright, I told myself.

For months we had Sunday afternoon meetings at our house. Doctors from a radius of ten or twelve miles came to join our discussions which were often enough vehement and angry. There was Parsons of Temple Martin who led the objectors, myself who spoke for Nye Bevan's Health Service, Ballard from Frampton who was open-minded and others including 'young' Jack Furlong who came to enjoy the argument.

Jack Furlong was like his father, a real man of Somerset, sportsman, lover of the country, broad of body and mind. He spoke with a slight engaging stammer. 'Well Ken, m'son, which way do we vo-vote today? I'm agin the government.' This and a roar of laughter would lighten the atmosphere and prevent us from taking ourselves too seriously. Jack's father, old Dr Furlong, had died during the war and my friendly battles with him were over, but Jack was a splendid replacement. He liked to pretend he had no brain but was in fact a shrewd as well as a lovable character. He had four children in about as many years and said to me one day, 'Me and the Missus, we 'ad four of 'em double quick, then someone tol-told us 'ow to stop 'em. We ain't 'ad no more.'

When we could get Jack Furlong to keep quiet the argument would go like this. Parsons always spoke first. 'We give our patients what they need,' he said. 'We are personally responsible for them. If they are not satisfied with us they can go somewhere else. Competition is essential to keep us on our toes. Take that away and we should degenerate into a lot of don't care nobodies, out of temper and out of date. What do you say, Ballard?'

'I'm the middle man so far. What do you think, Lane?'

'You talk about competition,' I said. 'Competition for what? It's competition for popularity. Anyone can be popular by stroking everyone in the right way, giving in to malingerers and putting on dramatic shows of treatment. Competition for popularity is no good, and competition to be the best doctor doesn't come into it, because most people don't know — have no way of knowing — a good doctor from a bad one, except an instinctive feeling about who they can trust. How popular do you get by telling a malingerer to go back to work? Competition for popularity is fundamentally wrong.'

'That was a long speech, m'son, and right all the way,' said Jack Furlong.

'Wait a minute.' Parsons again. 'You're saying that all doctors are crooks and all patients are fools. Most of us here are honest men, aren't we?' He looked round at the lounging figures blowing smoke rings or puffing at pipes. It was before the days when Drs Bradford and Hill had convinced us that smoking was about as beneficial to health as taking prussic acid. 'Aren't we?' he repeated.

'Of course we are, Tommy,' agreed Jack Furlong. 'Go on. You can talk longer than that.'

'Right then, we are all out for the good of our patients — their real good. If they need to be told straight out that they are killing themselves with drink we'll tell them so. If we think they are swinging the lead we'll tell them so. Patients by and large are a shrewd lot. They know when the doc is being honest and when he's pulling a fast one. Trust the patients, the great British public. They'll choose the best man and so keep us on our toes. Take away that competition and our standards will drop. With the best will in the world — we're all human — our standards will drop. And that's what's going to happen if we let Nye Bevan fool us into this health service.'

'That's better. Hear, hear,' said Jack Furlong.

Ballard pulled him up. 'It's all very well for you to make a joke of it, Jack, but this is a serious business. Our future and the future of the country depends on what we decide. Just be serious and tell us what you think yourself about it.'

'I can tell you that in about three words. It don't make a ha'porth of difference what-what you do one way or t'other.'

This took the wind out of our sails and there was a moment's silence, then Ballard, who was a solidly-built man, full of sound common sense, spoke words of moderation. 'Ideal doctors,' he said, 'will work any system but how good are we on the whole? Round here we are a pretty decent lot but what about some of the big towns and all the foreign doctors there are in practice? How do we get the best out of them? Isn't some form of competition necessary to keep them up to scratch?'

'I agree,' I said. 'You'd certainly cut out competition by a salaried service and I wouldn't agree to that. But you can get enough competition in any capitation system of payment. If patients are not satisfied with their doctors they can go to someone else, transfer like panel patients do now. So there would be moderate competition.'

'Then that's still competition for popularity,' put in one of the non-committed.

'It is,' I agreed. 'It's competition to give satisfaction to the patient but it's muted competition. In private practice, if you lose a patient it'll cost you several pounds a year. Under a capitation system, with a payment of say fifteen shillings a year per head, you would only lose that. Enough to make you safeguard your reputation as a whole, but not to be too obsessed with the need to please every patient.'

'I think you've got something there,' said Ballard. 'Partial competition is better than all-out competition for popularity. There's another thing. The N.H.S., if it comes, is optional. Anyone who doesn't want it can still be a private patient.'

'That means they have to pay twice over — once through taxes and once direct to the doctor.'

'There's another thing in favour of the N.H.S.,' I went on. 'It is to make a good service available to everyone.' I told them about my own childhood experience. 'Whether the patient can afford it or not they will have a right to a good service. That's the unanswerable argument.'

'Nonsense,' said Parsons. 'Which of us will make people pay if they can't afford it? The rich pay a guinea a visit and the poor get treated for nothing as often as not.'

'That's charity,' I told him. 'All very well for you but not very pleasant for the chap who simply can't afford to pay for his wife's long illness. He's got to accept charity and if he's proud he won't do it. The N.H.S. will give everyone the *right* to good treatment.'

'Hear, hear,' said Jack Furlong once more. He got up and added, 'Well, I'd better be off. Got an appointment at five.'

'The light's too bright for fishing, Jack. You won't catch anything tonight.'

'Want to take a bet?'

The arguments went on and the meetings became more friendly as time passed. In the end of course it was Jack Furlong who was right, in a way. Our deliberations made no apparent difference to the future, and when the new service was introduced on July 5th 1948 it was quickly accepted because it was a step in the right direction. But it was the power of public opinion that was decisive and we had played our minuscule part in its formation.

I have to admit that my own preoccupation that spring was with the size of practice I should find I had. The whole Pratt family to whom I had given enormous care left me at about that time. This was one cause of my shaken confidence. Another was the problem I had with possible malingerers.

My experience in the army was that whereas the great majority of the men would spurn any attempt at scrimshanking, there was often a minority who became a dead and dragging weight on the others. One attitude to these was that the unit was better without them, but this seemed unfair. It was the obvious duty of the doctors to spot them so that they could be made to serve in some department where they would do no harm to the fighting troops.

At home I was very keen — probably too keen — not to certify that men were ill when I believed they were fit for work. This decision is much more difficult than it sounds and excessive care over it can easily give you the reputation for never trusting your patients' word. My over-conscientiousness would certainly drive a lot of people away but it couldn't be helped.

My long battle with Stanley Barstow was a case in point.

In the autumn of 1946 he came to see me for the first time with back trouble. He had been seized with intense lumbar pain, he said, which spread down his right leg. It had come on suddenly as he got out of bed. His description of the difficulty of bending was vivid. He even had to kneel down to lift the lavatory seat.

I examined him and he was a clear-cut case of acute lumbago and sciatica. The fashionable diagnosis of pro-lapsed intervertebral disk had not yet arrived in Somerset, but this made no difference to the treatment which had been given for decades. Barstow had severe spasm of his lumbar muscles and a hint of a curve of the lower spine. There was an area of numbness over the outer side of his right leg, indicating sciatic nerve involvement. Any attempt to raise his straightened right leg when he lay flat on his back produced severe pain, whereas the left leg could be raised some forty degrees. When I let him relax after this test he remarked, 'Ah, that's better. Heaven that is when the pain eases a bit.'

He had all the classical signs and symptoms of acute lumbago and sciatic pain. 'I'm afraid you'll have to rest awhile,' I said.

'I hate being off work, Doctor,' he told me. 'The thought of all my buddies getting on with the job while I'm slacking here gets me down. Isn't there anything you can do to hurry it up?'

I had been shown some useful manipulations of the spine in the army and it suddenly struck me that this might be just the case to try my skill. There was a great deal of muscle spasm so I set to work very carefully. Gradually I managed to put his spine through a complete range of movement, especially in rotation. When I had finished he looked pleased. 'That's better,' he said. 'Not gone but a lot better.' He got up from his bed and walked gingerly round the room. 'Yes, it's a good bit better.'

I was delighted and told him to rest for a few days and to do some gentle exercises. I promised to visit him a week later.

To my surprise, on the morning I was due to visit him he turned up at the surgery. Most of the spasm had gone, the

135

curve in the spine had disappeared and the numbness in the right leg had completely cleared up. The pain was much better and he was already sleeping quite well again.

'I'll be right in a few days,' he said.

'I shouldn't hurry and you'd better be careful not to lift anything heavy for a time. And do those exercises several times a day.'

I was pleased with his progress and the evidence of my own prowess, and thought what a blessing it was to treat a man who genuinely wanted to get back to work.

He came again a week later and insisted that he was fit for work. All his symptoms had gone and the signs of trouble had completely disappeared. He thanked me profusely for what I had done and we parted in a glow of mutual respect and admiration.

In July 1947 he had a second attack almost exactly like the first. There was only one difference. The numbness on the right leg was not present this time. I did the same manipulation with the same improvement and left him to rest a few days as before.

On the Thursday of that week — my half-day — I went to see the cricket in Bath. I think Somerset were playing Gloucestershire and I arrived in the middle of the afternoon session. During the tea interval I took a walk round the ground to stretch my legs and who should I run into but Stanley Barstow. He was sitting in a wheelchair with a board supporting his back, having been pushed to the front of the crowd by sympathetic strangers.

We greeted each other like old friends. I had to admit I admired a man who was so keen on his cricket that he was prepared to come in a wheelchair to see his county play. I noted the supporting board with approval and asked him how he was. He seemed a little sheepish and said he hoped I didn't think he was doing anything to delay his recovery. My own thoughts were more concerned with the success of my manipulation than anything else.

This was his second attack so I had his spine and hips Xrayed. This showed nothing abnormal and after two weeks he came to see me quite recovered and ready for work. As I made my notes on his record card the wording was almost exactly the same as last time and suddenly this struck me as rather strange. My spinal manipulations had done no real good to any other patient, but they had worked like a charm with Stanley Barstow — twice. I supposed there might be some slight displacement of one of the intervertebral joints which the manipulation had fortunately corrected. All the same it was odd, and I was left with the suspicion that I had not quite reached the bottom of Stanley Barstow's trouble. He was such a model patient that I trusted him implicitly.

He had his third attack in November 1947 when events repeated themselves precisely. The signs were exactly the same, still without the numbness of the right leg. This time I began to wonder if I had got my assessment of the case wrong. Lumbar pain was, after all, the easiest of all conditions to exaggerate or to simulate. It was the lead-swinger's trump card and very difficult to deny. Stanley Barstow had produced such text-book supporting signs and symptoms, and was so graphic in his descriptions, that the thought that he might be deceiving me had never before entered my head, but now I wasn't so sure.

For the first time I looked carefully at his expression and appearance. His hair was always heavily oiled and firmly plastered down on his head. His nose was small and his expression almost unnaturally benign. I wondered, and the small shadows of doubt began to grow.

I told him I was concerned about his repeated attacks and would like Dr Wyburn to see him.

'But I'm nearly right now,' he said.

'I know, but when will you get another attack?'

Wyburn examined him carefully, confirmed the muscle spasm and the evidence of recovering sciatic nerve irritation. He could offer no real help but added, 'I'm not sure I would trust that man.'

So the doubts went on.

This attack lasted longer than the others but after three weeks he said he was fit for work again. He thanked me profusely, said he didn't know what he would do without my manipulations, and left with his signing-off certificate.

My mind went back over the details of his case. Was it really possible that a man could possess himself of such accurate knowledge of the signs and symptoms of a disease and then be a good enough actor to deceive me completely?

There was the lumbar muscle spasm — well, that could be put on. There was the slight curve of the spine in the attacks which disappeared when he recovered. This would be more difficult but could perhaps be assumed. There was the pain on raising the right leg from the lying position. This could be simulated. The numbness of the leg as though the sciatic nerve was under pressure was concrete evidence of organic trouble. Taking the case as a whole, no one was likely to know all the exact signs and symptoms of root pressure on the sciatic nerve, and even if they did it would be very painful to pretend to numbness of the leg that didn't exist. My pinpricks had been very sharp and he hadn't winced.

Then I remembered that this one convincing sign had disappeared after the first attack. Could this possibly mean that it had been simulated but had been too painful to do a second time? The sharp pricks which he had denied feeling might have troubled him enough to make him give up that particular piece of evidence.

He had had one attack during Bath cricket week, but people did get ill during cricket week so that was no evidence either way.

I thought again about my manipulations. They had been very gentle and I had used no sudden force. There had been no snick as of a bone slipping into place or adhesions being divided. Had they really been so remarkably effective?

When he developed his fourth attack in May 1948 I was really puzzled. Attacks of such severity which left no residual abnormality were difficult to understand. I discussed the problem with Tom Wyburn again.

'How much time has he had away from work altogether?' he asked.

I produced his record card and added up the times on sick leave.

'He had a total of five weeks in 1946,' I said, 'but that includes three weeks with bronchitis in May that year. Then he's had —' I added the weeks carefully from the scribbled A's, C's and C offs on the card. 'He's had five weeks in 1947, all with back trouble.'

'Any significance in that or just coincidence,' Wyburn pondered.

'Not much evidence in itself but I wonder —'

Two days after I had given him his certificate of incapacity that May I called at his house unexpectedly. There was some delay before I was admitted, but when I went into their sitting-room Barstow was lying on the floor. I had told him this was a good position and he could lie down whenever he felt like it.

His wife appeared to be decorating the kitchen but was dressed quite smartly while Barstow was in his shirt-sleeves. I stood over him and talked for a while and before I left I noticed a spot of paint on his hand.

'Tried to have a go myself just now,' he said. 'Thought I could stand up and do a bit but it's no good.'

He knew by this time that he was under suspicion but showed not the slightest resentment. Most people respond angrily to any suggestion that they are not being genuine, but not Stanley Barstow. He smiled in sublime confidence. Either he was entirely innocent or he knew he had the doctors beaten.

That evening I got out his record once more. There must be a clue somewhere, as by then I was convinced he was malingering. Suddenly a possibility struck me. There was little to be gained by pretending to be ill when he wasn't unless there was some money in it somewhere. His panel payment for incapacity together with his club money would hardly equal his normal earnings.

I telephoned the factory where he worked and spoke to the personnel manager. I asked whether they paid their employees when they were on sick leave. 'We allow them twenty-five days paid sick leave each year,' he said.

'You are very generous,' I told him. 'So your people are much better off sick than working for those twenty-five days — five weeks in fact. Their sick pay is not taxed and they have full pay as well.'

'That's right.'

Barstow was well on the way to his third period of five weeks sick leave in three successive years. One spring he had been off sick with bronchitis for three weeks and that year his back trouble had lasted a correspondingly shorter time. Evidently he would wait till nearly the end of each year and then take enough sick leave to make up a total of five weeks. As he knew he would be 'ill' for five weeks each year it seemed only reasonable to make one of the weeks coincide with cricket week.

I made up my mind that next time I saw him I would have some sort of a showdown with him. He came to the surgery at the end of a week's sick leave and I began, 'I'm afraid I've been wrong about you all this time. You've had exactly five weeks sick leave each year. Is this because you have five weeks paid sick leave from your firm each year?'

For a moment he had the grace to look startled. 'I don't understand,' he said.

'I think you do. There is one way of making sure. Strip off your shirt, will you?'

I examined his back carefully, pressing hard on each spinal process from mid-dorsal region downwards. 'No pain?' I asked.

'No, nothing much.'

Then I made a great show of examining his right calf, finally squeezing it firmly. 'Still no pain?'

'No, not really.'

'Dress up, will you?'

I wrote out a signing-off certificate. 'You haven't had back trouble at all, have you? You've been malingering.'

I looked straight at him. I had bargained on making him think I had positive evidence that his back was normal and that there was one definite sign of lumbago that was missing because he hadn't been told about it. The gamble worked and he made no reply. There were no fireworks, no angry denials, no violent scenes. He looked at me as if to say 'you've been a long time finding that out' and accepted a signing-off note. I was left feeling curiously deflated.

It was the end of May 1948 and the new National Health Service was due to be introduced in five weeks time. Patients on our panel list would be transferred automatically to our N.H.S. list, but every other man woman and child would receive a card which they had to sign and take to the doctor of their choice. These were to be sent by the doctors to the administrators, and a fixed payment would be made each quarter to the doctor concerned for every patient on his list.

During the first week in June I received about 150 cards and in the second week about 300. With my panel list of 1,200 there was a long way to go before I had the number I had hoped for. To maintain my present income I should need about 2,700 patients.

In the middle of June I received notification that some twenty of my panel patients had applied to be taken off my list. This was a considerable shock and when I discovered that all of them worked at the same factory as Stanley Barstow I became angry. For a man to engage in a battle of wits with me was slightly funny, but to slander me to his friends was beyond forgiveness. When more transfers were notified during the next week I became somewhat paranoid. There was nothing I could do about it. There was and is no punishment for malingering, and any patient is free to malign his doctor.

A drop of a hundred or so patients on my list could be sustained, but more than this would mean financial hardship unless we took the two older children away from school. This I would not do unless it became essential.

I told myself that I must be prepared to have only about 2,300 patients on my N.H.S. list. Provided Wyburn and the other partners kept their lists well up things might not be too bad, but I was well prepared for some degree of humiliation.

Towards the end of June cards came in in floods and I began to hope all would be well. When my final list became available on July 5th 1948 I found I had over 3,400 patients on my list.

When the flurry of anxiety was over I began to wonder whether after all I had been wrong about Stanley Barstow.

If he had in fact been genuinely ill he would have been justified in giving me a bad name. I had no idea which doctor he had transferred to, so it was impossible to ask his opinion. The case solved itself a year later.

I went to see Somerset playing Kent in Bath and there, as large as life, was Stanley Barstow. He was sitting in a wheelchair in front of the crowd, enjoying a fine view of the match.

'Well Barstow,' I greeted him, 'you are still in the same state as before, are you?'

'Exactly the same,' he replied. 'Dr Parsons doesn't agree with your opinion.'

'Evidently not,' I said and left him.

He had not risked transferring to one of the Melbrook doctors whom I met daily in the hospital for fear of my telling them my experience. Now he had inadvertently let me know who was attending him. Even if Dr Parsons found him out in a year or so he would have robbed his firm and the country of a considerable sum of money. And he would have been quite safe as that form of robbery is never punished.

After some thought I telephoned Parsons and told him of my experience with Barstow. He blustered a little at first but took my opinion seriously. When I met him some time later he had made up his mind and expressed his opinion in very strong language.

'I called on him, you know,' he said, 'after you rang me up. I live a long way away from him and he wasn't expecting me. Do you know what he was doing?'

'Decorating the kitchen?'

'On the fourth day of his sick leave he was building a wall in his garden.'

'What did you do?'

'I put the fear of God into him. Told him he would hear from the Ministry of Health and gave him a signing-off certificate. Pity there is no punishment for that sort of fraud but he won't do it again.'

'Not with you or me, anyway,' I said.

12

It has been said that we must learn to weep before we can laugh. In the case of Simon and Sally Burdon the tears certainly came before the laughter.

Sally Burdon was not a jolly person but she was a woman of solid character, healthy and attractive. She and Simon had been married for five or six years and had two children. She had a good university degree and had taught modern languages before she was married. Simon was a successful executive in a firm in the city. They lived in a fine house in the country which combined the character of age with all the convenience of modernisation. Few people had swimming-pools in those days, but they had a hard tennis court and some two acres of garden and orchard. They were both keen tennis players and there were week-end tennis parties for much of the year. They seemed to have everything.

One day Sally brought young Edmond, the older child, to the surgery. He had a lot of catarrh, enough to make him bubble and squeak like an old bronchitic, but he seemed remarkably well in himself. I examined him but concluded that he needed no treatment except exercise in the fresh air which would help him to cough up the offending mucus. I told Sally what I thought.

'Can't you give him something to clear this awful catarrh? Some penicillin or something?'

In those days we gave penicillin when it was needed and not when a spontaneous cure was a virtual certainty. I told her that he needed no medicine.

She looked annoyed. 'He's driving Simon mad,' she said, 'and look at him. His nose is running like that all the time.'

'Yes, he certainly needs plenty of handkerchiefs.' I smiled at her but it was no use.

'Couldn't I have some cough medicine — just to show Simon that I've done my best to get help?'

'Yes, of course.' I wrote a prescription and repeated that with fresh air his nose would clear in a few days.

'You mean the medicine is no good really?' Her manner was resentful and this was unlike her.

'It will do Simon good.' I smiled again but could get no response. This was when I ought to have sat back in my chair and brought the conversation round to herself in the hope of finding out whether anything was wrong with her. I didn't and she departed, leaving a strong atmosphere of dissatisfaction behind her.

It must have been a week or ten days later that she came to see me again, not with Edmond this time but with Harriet, the younger child, aged two. Harriet was sleeping badly — late teething according to her mother. She would wake and scream in the early hours of the morning and again she was 'driving Simon mad'. I examined her and found nothing wrong but was persuaded to prescribe a few doses of mild sedative.

Ten days later Edmond was brought to see me again. This time he had started bedwetting at the age of three and a half. It was then, at last, that I began to ask myself whether all was well in the home.

The Burdons must have been one of the first families to make me realise that children were often only ill because there was something wrong with the parents. So after I had suggested the then fashionable treatment for bedwetting I asked Sally about herself. She was looking tired and depressed.

'Do you have any help with the children?' I asked her.

'Why should I? I'm quite capable of looking after them myself.'

I sat and looked at her with what was meant to be an expression of sympathy. 'Quite capable,' she repeated briskly but this time there was a catch in her voice.

I waited and presently she went on, 'Besides, they are my main consolation at present.'

144

So there *was* something else wrong. I suppose my manner must have become more encouraging because she suddenly came out of the shell that had seemed to envelop her.

'Yes,' she said, 'something is badly wrong. Our marriage is breaking up.'

This, in those days, was nothing short of a bombshell. Marriages in the country didn't break up. They might go through difficult times but they didn't break up. By this time I was very much concerned. I knew them well. They had always appeared a very happy couple, well suited to each other, endowed with every possible blessing — health, children, money, interesting work and plenty of friends. 'What's gone wrong?' I asked.

At last the words poured out of her. 'It's utterly mad but Simon and I are hardly on speaking terms. It all started two months ago when we had a mild ordinary row over something or other, but instead of making it up it's gone from bad to worse and I don't know why. Sometimes we seem to hate each other. As to sleeping together it's out of the question. We've been in separate rooms for weeks and each of us blames the other. Simon says I've changed, that I've got hard and think of nothing but the children, that I'm selfish, have no sense of humour and as a last straw that I don't attract him any more.'

'And what do you say to him?'

'That he's changed too, that's all.'

'It sounds like an ordinary quarrel. It can't last, surely?'

'An ordinary quarrel lasting two months?'

'Neither of you have been attracted by anyone else?'

'No, I certainly haven't. And I'm sure I'd know if Simon had. I'm sure there's no one else.'

'Then how can he keep away from your bed?'

'I don't know unless he's got something wrong with him.' And here the solid mature Sally Burdon began to cry.

'Could you persuade him to come and see me,' I said. 'I could make sure he is physically alright and perhaps have a talk with him at the same time.'

'I'll try but I don't think he'll come.'

Young Edmond was getting more restless every minute,

running round the room, investigating cupboards and generally distracting my attention. Sally was too distressed to notice him. When he began waving a vaginal speculum in the air I stood up and took it from him. 'Try and persuade Simon to come and see me at the weekend. Tell him you've made an appointment with me. Then come down yourself a day or two later. Get someone to look after the children for an hour so that we can have time to talk. I can't imagine that a good marriage like yours can really break down. You are well in yourself, aren't you?'

'I suppose so, yes. I'm miserably depressed, that's all.'

To my surprise Simon came to see me. 'There's nothing wrong with me,' he said, 'but for the sake of peace in the house I've come to see you as ordered.' He sat back looking at me as though that concluded the medical part of the interview, and we might as well talk about something else.

'Sally seemed to be seriously worried about you,' I told him.

'Worried about me?' he repeated. 'I don't think that's very likely.'

'There were tears anyway.'

'Oh yes, plenty of tears. We've had plenty of tears lately.' I waited for him to go on. 'She's completely changed this last month or two. Seems to have lost all interest in me.'

'Am I going to examine you?'

'Just as you please. There's nothing the matter with me.'

I took his blood pressure and tested his urine. Early diabetes might have affected his sex life but there was nothing wrong.

'I wish I could help you. How did it all start?'

'God knows. One of those idiotic rows that normally blow over as soon as the woman in the case feels better. You know what I mean. But this time Sally has gone on being withdrawn, behaving as though she's either indifferent to me or positively dislikes me.'

'It's not always the woman, you know. We have our aggressions too and they seem to need an airing every now and then. But that's all normal enough. There must be some reason for this going on so long.'

'I've come to the conclusion she's basically selfish and now when she's having a bit of trouble with the children she's not liking it.'

'I gather neither of you have got anyone else?'

'No, not yet. But if things go on like this I won't vouch for anything.'

'Have you made any efforts to make it up?'

'Good heavens yes. I've been to her room over and over again at night, sat on her bed and tried to make it up. Let's face it, she's a very attractive girl. But she won't budge. Says I'm only interested in sex. Well of course I'm interested in sex. She wouldn't like it if I weren't but it's not my sole preoccupation.'

Recording the various conversations as well as I can remember them — and they may be coloured by hindsight — I am amazed that I didn't spot the cause of the trouble. But of course I didn't know then what is common knowledge now.

I was puzzled. I was no expert in marriage guidance. My usual method was to try to explain each to the other and then tell each party that the other was very much in love with them. Not very scientific but it often worked. I knew the two of them — Sally and Simon — quite well socially as well as professionally and they were a pleasant extroverted couple, easy-going and sensible. It was hard to imagine how they had got bogged down in a long quarrel like this.

'There's no sexual problem on either side?'

'Never has been. We've always been fine together.'

'What is your actual criticism of Sally? You said she was basically selfish.'

'Well that's not true really. She's marvellous with the kids, never complains however many times she has to get up to them at night. No, she's not really selfish. She just behaves as though she is tired of me and that's all there is to it.'

'And she thinks you are tired of her. Well, one or other of you has got to put your pride in your pocket and say you are sorry.'

'Sorry for what?'

'I suppose you've both said some pretty nasty things about each other? Tried to hurt the other to produce a reaction?'

'I suppose so.'

'Well, say you're sorry and mean it. Then she'll say she's sorry and it might be all over.'

'Not a chance. It might have worked the first day or so but we've got too entrenched now.'

'You are both seeing only the worst side of each other. You haven't any real complaint except that she's stopped being as loving as usual.'

'O.K., I'll try again. Thanks for your help. I never knew this was doctor's business.'

'Of course it is. We're interested in preventive medicine. This sort of thing can make either or both of you ill. Choose a careful moment and say you're sorry and see what happens. Give her a large gin first.'

'Good idea that, anyway.'

But of course it didn't work.

Sally came to see me again a few days later. 'You must have told Simon to say he was sorry but he obviously didn't mean it. He's changed and we simply don't like each other any more. If it weren't for the children we'd get a divorce.'

I wanted to knock their heads together. They had everything and still wanted and needed each other, yet at the first hint of aggression or antagonism in each other they talked of divorce.

I let her run on for a while but it was the same story. They had both 'changed' and didn't like what they saw of each other.

'Now listen to me Sally,' I said, 'you are behaving like a couple of children. Of course your characters haven't changed all of a sudden. You are the same people who lived together perfectly happily for several years. You've quarrelled and are both seeing the worst side of each other. There is a bad side in all of us. When anyone seems too nice, too kind and unselfish, I say to myself, where's the baddie beneath the goodie? Don't you know what I mean? We all have aggressions. We'd be spineless and colourless if we hadn't. We all have bad patches, but when you live with someone you've got to take the good with the bad. There is plenty of good in you two. You are a splendid mother and housekeeper and you do a lot in the village over there. You should hear how people talk about you. And Simon is a very good fellow — utterly faithful to you although he must be very attractive to women. He wants you very badly, I can tell you that, but he feels you have changed and don't want him any more. Don't you think you ought to be grateful for what you've got?'

'You don't understand,' she said with ominous calm. 'We are neither of us doing anything terribly wrong but we are not interested in each other any more.'

I was out of my depth and we got nowhere. I began to feel frustrated and angry, but if they insisted on torturing each other there was nothing more I could do about it.

I met Jack Furlong in the hospital after this last interview and without mentioning names blurted out the whole infuriating story to him. 'Tell 'un to get in bed with her and m-m-make her, that's the ans-answer.'

Jack had a happy marriage but not, I imagine, by reason of this kind of therapy. He and his wife accepted each other as they really were.

I talked to Jessica about the Burdons that evening. Her solution was equally simplistic. 'They've got too much money,' she said. 'If they had to plan together to buy another chair or a carpet when they could afford it, like we did at that stage, it would do them good.'

Saving and buying is certainly a pleasant shared occupation but this couldn't be the whole trouble.

During the next few weeks I saw Sally several times with one or other of the children. They seemed to be afflicted with continual colds, bilious attacks, bedwetting and peevishness. It was more and more obvious that their health was suffering because of the atmosphere in the house. I told Sally this and asked again whether there was any hope of their being reconciled.

'None whatever,' she said. 'We made it up for one night and slept together but next day it was the same as ever. It's gone too far now. We've just got to put up with it.'

The final phase of the Burdon story began one Sunday evening. Sally phoned me and said rather coldly, 'Simon says he's got a pain in his stomach.' Not that he had a pain but that he 'said he had a pain'.

'How long?' I asked.

'He's been complaining all day but I told him to wait till tomorrow. It might be better by then. But now he says he thinks it is something bad and he can't wait. I don't expect it's anything.'

I went over to see him and he had an acute appendix with a thirty-six-hour history. He was in real trouble and might already have perforated so I arranged for an ambulance to take him in to the city hospital straight away. Under the National Health Service the age of the general practitioner surgeon was rapidly dying and Tom Wyburn was no longer doing our surgery. It was a welcome relief to be able to shed the responsibility of a case like this at once.

When the ambulance had taken Simon away I talked to Sally. I wondered whether she was really as hard-boiled as she sounded, or whether this emergency was not just the thing to bring them to their senses — the equivalent of having their heads knocked together.

I was annoyed with her for delaying so long before she sent for me and told her she should have known better.

She looked distressed but spoke defensively. 'He's always complaining lately. He sleeps in another room and I didn't know till this morning that he had had a bad night. Then he said he was a bit better and ate a little breakfast. He's pretty tough and got up at lunch-time. I thought he was getting better. Anyway you apparently told him that our state of misery might make either of us ill.' The accusing look was only half-veiled.

'Did he vomit?' I asked.

'He said he did in the night.'

'Didn't you realise that must mean something?'

'Well, no. Anyone can be sick.'

'Sally, don't you see you are being much too hard on Simon? You really must look at the way you are behaving to him. He's been very ill for thirty-six hours. He ought to have been operated on in the night or at least early this morning. His appendix may well have ruptured and set up peritonitis.'

Perhaps I was being unkind to rub it in, but I felt she had been neglectful and told her so. Had I known what was to follow I would not have been so openly critical, but in the back of my mind was the thought that once she felt a little guilt her manner to Simon might soften.

Simon was operated on that evening. He had not perforated and all seemed well. Just as I got to bed, a little before midnight, a very agitated Sally telephoned me. She was overcome by remorse and in great need of comfort and reassurance.

'I'm feeling so worried,' she said. 'You told me I had neglected him. Will he be alright?'

'Yes, of course he will. He hadn't perforated so he ought to be quite straightforward. I rang the surgeon and he seemed satisfied with him. Stop worrying and get some sleep.'

This, I thought, will surely be the end of their estrangement. It was, but not in the way I thought.

On the Thursday of that week, my half-day, I did my usual visit to the city hospital to see any of my patients who were there. Simon was well and very cheerful. 'I'm hoping this will do the trick,' he said, 'between Sally and me, I mean.'

'I'm afraid I was rather brutal with her on Sunday night after you went off,' I replied. 'I told her she ought to have sent for me much sooner.'

'That wasn't her fault. I didn't get her up in the night. I thought it was some mushrooms I'd eaten. It wasn't till the Sunday evening that I knew there was something really wrong. Then she sent straight away. I hope you didn't put the wind up her too much.'

'I hope not. Perhaps I was a bit harsh though.' It was good to hear Simon sticking up for her and I had high hopes that the worst of their troubles were over.

It was on the following Saturday evening that the bombshell exploded. I met one of the Burdons' neighbours in the town. 'Bad job about poor old Simon Burdon,' he said.

'Being in hospital, you mean?' Even as I spoke I felt a sense of apprehension.

'He's dead. They rang Sally this morning. Didn't you know? Died this morning.'

I was shocked as I have seldom been in my life. He must have had an embolus — still a risk even in ideal conditions.

I went straight over to see Sally. On the way I was horribly aware of my own clumsiness in telling her that she had neglected him. Poor girl, how would she ever live that down?

She was of course completely shattered and I had no idea what to say. A neighbour was looking after the children who were quite unaffected by the news. The indifference of children to a tragedy they will only understand much later always seems to make these situations more poignant.

'When did it happen?' I asked Sally.

'Early this morning. They rang me at eight o'clock. I can't believe it. He was so well yesterday.' Her face was pale and she looked ten years older than a week earlier. Her eyes were red with crying, her nose was shining and she seemed to have shrunk in size. She sat mopping her face and eyes, then sobbed. 'And it was my fault. I ought to have sent for you sooner. You said so. I can't believe it.' Her voice trailed off. I sat opposite her, sharing her misery and not without a worrying sense of guilt myself.

'It was not your fault, Sally. You must get that clearly into your head.'

'What does it matter now anyway?'

I have seen much grief in my life but none more intense than this. I had to go on talking. 'His appendix was removed in good time and he ought not to have died. So you hadn't delayed it too long. You hadn't. I don't know what happened. He may have had an embolism — a clot that moves into the lung. I don't know. I'll find out about it.'

Presently she was able to talk again. 'I think I must have made him ill. He kept trying to make it up but I couldn't. I seemed to be possessed, bewitched or something. Then in hospital we were both feeling different. I hoped when he came home —'

The household seemed to have been blasted by the news.

It was unnaturally silent, as though there was already a dead body in the bedroom upstairs.

I left her after half an hour or so with some sedative tablets that I thought might help the worst of the shock. Driving home I had the leaden feeling I had only experienced once before, when my young assistant was drowned in Blagdon Lake in 1940.

As soon as I got home I telephoned the city hospital and was put through to the ward Simon had been in. I asked for Sister and when she came on the line I said, 'Can you tell me what happened to Mr Burdon, the acute appendix, Simon Burdon?'

'Nothing's happened to him, Doctor. He's sitting here playing cards.'

For the second time that day I couldn't believe my ears. I was stunned. 'Are you there, Doctor?' said the phone. I pulled myself together with an effort.

'His wife had a message from the hospital this morning to say he was dead.'

'Dead? Whoever told her that? He's doing splendidly.'

'What a relief. We've got it right now, haven't we? Simon Burdon with an acute appendix is doing quite well?'

A cheerful laugh at the other end reassured me. 'Yes, that's quite right.'

'I'll telephone his wife and tell her there's been a mistake. I left her only a few minutes ago — shattered by what she was told this morning.'

'I can't think what happened. I'll go straight down to the office and find out. You will deal with Mrs Burdon?' There was a pause, then, 'No, it's alright, Mr Burdon. There's been a misunderstanding, that's all. Your wife is perfectly alright.'

I heard Simon's voice asking, 'Who's that on the phone?' and Sister told him. 'May I speak to him?' Simon said and a moment later he was on the line.

I was still somewhat shaken. I told him that Sally had been given a false report that he had died.

'Then I'm going straight home,' Simon said.

'Talk to her on the phone in five minutes,' I told him.

153

'Just give me time to tell her you are alright.'

Sister phoned me a few minutes later with the explanation of the mistake. Another Mr S. Burdon — a very old man — had died in the night and the office had informed the wrong relative.

This curious mistake happened only once in my whole working life. Indeed I have never heard of another such case but it was enough to provide a very traumatic experience.

Simon insisted on being discharged the next day and the Burdons' domestic troubles were over. When I saw them together on the Monday they were like a couple of honeymooners. Both were profoundly sobered for a day or two but there was no more estrangement.

I called on them again a week or two later and the whole family were sitting in the garden. The children — both naked — were playing with a spray from the garden hose and the scene is vivid in my memory. Young Edmond began to shout with laughter and his sister followed suit. Both parents echoed them and finally I caught the infection myself and we were all laughing. For a few seconds the place rang with the sound of carefree laughter.

Children respond with incredible speed by illness or happiness to the atmosphere of the home. In this case their behaviour was like a flag hoisted high to indicate that all was now well.

I was puzzled for a long time over the three-month estrangement between two people who had made a good marriage. In time the cause became perfectly obvious.

It was not that they had too much luxury, too much of everything.

It was not even that they failed to realise that we all have our aggressions, our unpleasant side, that we are all 'miserable sinners' and must accept each other as we are. It was something much more simple.

Some years later Sally had a mild attack of endogenous depression and I realised that a similar attack had been the cause of the earlier trouble between them. Undiagnosed depression — either endogenous or post-puerperal — is now a well recognised cause of marital breakdown. The sparkle, the fun, the vitality in one of a couple disappears through no fault of their own. What more natural than that the other should think their spouse has changed, lost interest, fallen out of love. And change in one induces change in the other. The solution to the problem is so easy once you know the answer. Fortunately nowadays the condition is eminently treatable.

It is not fanciful to suggest that the false report of Simon's death represented the shock treatment that sometimes cures depression. I think it did.

And had there been no shock? The depression might have lasted many months, or on the other hand I might have recognised and treated it when others had reported a similar experience.

'The art,' as Hippocrates said, indeed 'takes so long to learn.'

13

Albert Randall was not only one of the hardest workers I ever knew, he was, joy of joys, a character.

To begin with he was some six feet six inches tall, broad in proportion and enormously strong. He was a repair worker at the pits and therefore often on night shift. In his spare time he ran a smallholding of something over an acre and on this he bred pigs, kept a multitude of hens and a cow as well as a fruit and vegetable garden. The hens were in a literal sense 'free range'. They ranged across the fields round the Randalls' house and often enough into the neighbours' gardens — even occasionally into their houses. The boundary of the holding was a dry stone wall about four feet high and this of course the hens took at their leisure.

Fortunately none of the neighbours were obsessional gardeners and no one seemed to worry about the trespass. I believe they all had their eggs from Mrs Randall at a low price and when a pig was killed the bacon was shared too. It was a pleasant cooperative society in which most of the work was done by Albert, with a free hand from a neighbour whenever it was called for. Albert was the uncrowned king of the little community, respected for his character and loved for his generosity.

I remember being told a long story by one of his elderly neighbours about how he had dealt with two marauding teenagers whom he caught stealing his pears.

'Them two younguns,' said old Parsons, 'clambered over Alby's wall one night an' zet about them pears. Twas thic tree at th'end yonder and they'm zlow ter ripen, zee? Twas middle October an' Alby useter watch them pears

every day gettin' yellerer and zarfter, yellerer an' zarfter.'
The description of the luscious pears was so vivid that I
swear he had to stop because his mouth was watering.
'Delicious them pears,' he said, 'ah. Well, that evenin',
twer gettin' dusk at the toime, an' these younguns did get
in, zee? They'd 'elped theirzelves to 'alf a dozen when out
come Alby wi' a roar you could 'ave 'eered over Mendip to
Wells, Oi reckon. Neow they was biggish lads — vufteen
or zuxteen mebbe, an' they was a bit zmart loike at vurzt.

"Wot be yeou young zkunks doin' wi' my pears?" says
Alby. "Come on, 'and 'em ower or Oi'll beat the 'ides orf
yer."

'Well, one on 'em were a mort vresh loike an' 'er zaid
yeou can zpare a vew on 'em, Guvner, er zaid.

There was a pause to impress the drama of the event
then the old man went on, 'Well, Alby looked at 'un. 'E
looked at 'un. An' then thic youngun 'e larfed. 'E larfed.'
Another impressive pause. Old Parsons was happy reliv-
ing that October evening and a smile settled on his
wrinkled old face. For a moment I thought he was going to
forget to finish the tale, but not he.

'Zo Alby 'e ups an' zpreads out 'is girt arms, 'e does.'
He illustrated by stretching out his rheumaticky shoulders
to the limit. 'Then 'er ketched 'old on one on 'em in one
'and, an' t'other in t'other 'and, an' er grups 'em round
the necks loike a couple o' chicken — an' lifts 'em up in the
air. Then 'er walks as zlow an' calm as if 'e were in church,
carryin' them younguns ower to yon wall, an' 'e zwings
vust one then t'other ower the wall an' drarps 'em into thic
bed o' ztinger nettles. Yeou should 'uv 'eered them 'oller.
Then 'er ztood there lookin' at 'em. Never zaid a wurd,
jus' looked at 'em. Ah, oh, ah.' And he dissolved into a
happy chuckle.

This gives some idea of Albert Randall's muscle power,
but he was a gentle giant. He was on my list of patients but
I didn't treat him for years. When I called to see his wife or
one of the children, I enjoyed not so much a chat, more a
quiet communication with him.

The outbuildings on Albert's smallholding were a
hybrid collection of sheds made partly of wood and partly

157

of galvanised iron. The biggest of these, where the cow was kept in winter, had an upper storey which harboured animal foods, some straw and some hay. One day the roof of this building needed repair; a sheet of galvanised iron had rusted badly and had to be replaced. As often happened the work was undertaken by one of the neighbours. Len Parsons — a young fellow just married — brought his ladder over one Saturday afternoon and set about the simple job with every evidence of enthusiasm. His young bride came with him and somehow they must have become too light-hearted because Len fell off the ladder. It was an awkward fall of ten or twelve feet and he landed badly. Somehow or other he struck his hand on a jagged piece of old galvanised iron and dislocated his shoulder at the same time. The hand bled badly from a severed artery and the dislocated shoulder made control of this somewhat difficult.

The next thing that happened — also before my arrival on the scene — was that young Leonard's wife fainted at the sight of so much of her husband's blood spurting on to the ground.

Alby was of course deeply distressed and for a few minutes was convinced he had, or soon would have, a couple of corpses on his hands. I was welcomed as the saviour of the situation and led hurriedly along the path to the scene of the disaster.

It seemed likely that the young woman had only fainted — she was sipping water when I got there — but the hand was still pulsating blood on to what looked like the floor of a slaughter-house. Alby was gripping the forearm but having no effect on the bleeding. Young Leonard Parsons was looking very pale, partly from shock and partly from loss of blood.

There was no time to talk and after a brief glance at the torn hand I pressed a pad of lint on to the spurting artery and bound it up. I let him lie still for a few minutes while I took a look at his wife. Unhurt, she was in the wretched but safe state of recovering from a faint.

Leonard was not unnaturally feeling faint too, partly from pain in his dislocated shoulder. It was worthwhile trying to reduce the dislocation on the spot because this is often easy — especially when the muscles are relaxed by shock. Three times out of four the reduction can be done by the family doctor; the fourth case will often tax the skill of an orthopaedic specialist. As it turned out, with routine manipulation the shoulder slipped back into position more smoothly than usual and relief of pain was immediate.

'Thank God you was quick, zir,' said Alby. 'When a pig bleeds like yon 'e's soon gone. Oi reckoned young Len were a gonner as well as 'is missus.'

'If that ever happens again Alby,' I told him, 'press firmly on the bleeding spot and you'll usually stop it.'

'Ah,' said Alby, 'Oi should er knowed. Were a bit zcared loike. Wi' 'is new missus lookin' loike dead Oi were prarper zcared, Oi can tell 'ee. If Oi could er done wot yeou did, Oi could er zaved un a mort o' blood.'

'He'll be alright,' I told him, 'and you'll know next time.'

'Would Oi arve the nerve zir? Oi can vace trouble in the pits an' Oi can vace trouble with the animals but Oi'd need ter know a deal more to dare touch zummon loike 'e were.'

By good fortune both young Parsons and his wife rapidly began to look better, and this added a touch of drama to my ministrations. I didn't realise till a week or two later how deeply Alby had been impressed.

The cottage hospital was less than a mile away and I ran young Leonard up there in my car. His wife was very insistent about coming with us and promised not to faint again — for what such a promise was worth. I clamped the spurting artery under local anaesthesia and with a few stitches he was soon nearly as good as new.

This was one of the occasions when treatment was easy, successful and rewarding. Too often in an accident all the family doctor can do is to pack the casualties off to a major hospital, and this gives him little satisfaction. I am not however recording this case for that reason, but because of what followed in my long relationship with Alby Randall.

For several years after the war — until I had a junior

partner to help me — I lectured to the St John Ambulance Brigade every other Friday evening. Either 'the Super' — Superintendent Fleetwood — or his assistant, Sergeant Paragon, would be in charge. Fleetwood was in charge of first aid treatment at the colliery. He was a good practical teacher of first aid and a good but effortless disciplinarian. Paragon was a strict but not an effortless disciplinarian. He was a small man with a Stentorian voice who exerted all his powers to dominate the somewhat rustic assembly.

One evening a new member turned up at our meeting. It was none other than Albert Randall and within a few minutes of his joining us, it was evident that between him and Sergeant Paragon sparks would fly.

There was always a short drill session before our lectures and exercises, and this was where Paragon came into his own.

Albert Randall stood several inches above the tallest of the other members and was inclined to move slowly. Being a miner he had not been in the services during the war, and to put it mildly drill didn't come naturally to him. His right turn was a shuffle several seconds after everyone else and when it came to marching round the room he took one step for everyone else's one and three-quarters.

I am not sure whether Paragon was disconcerted or utterly delighted at the prospect of being allowed in the course of duty to shout non-stop at such a large man as Albert Randall. But he had met his match.

'Quick march, left right, left right, now Randall keep step, left right.' He walked up to Randall, shouting in his ear and stamping as he did so.

Very soon Albert Randall had had enough. He strolled out of line, folded his arms and stood looking placidly down at the ferocious face of Sergeant Paragon.

'Get back in line Randall,' Paragon shouted.

'I ain't come 'ere ter be shouted at by the loikes of yeou, Harry,' Randall replied. ''Twas ter learn vust aid Oi did come. Bain't thic wot we'm 'ere vor?'

'You'll get no instruction till you'm done yer drill. Get back in line, wull 'e?'

But Albert strolled over to a chair, sat down with hands on knees waiting for the next move — which as the senior officer present was clearly up to me.

I sympathised with him but it was impossible to do away, for his sake, with the time-honoured two minutes drill before the practical training. I always regarded spit and polish to be alright in its place, but as an aid to the acquisition of medical or surgical skills to be superfluous. Because of my feelings in this matter I firmly refused to wear the uniform of Divisional Surgeon in the St John Ambulance Brigade, and I was not the one to insist on the importance of drill. The men must be smart on any public duty, I agreed, but my job was to teach them practical first aid. The drill was for others. My lack of logic can be shot to pieces of course, but the men put up with my stubbornness for many years. I was fond of each one of them and will never forget their absolute reliability during the first years of the war.

'I'm afraid Sergeant Paragon is right,' I told Randall. 'There is always a short drill before the lecture. Stay this evening and see how you like the teaching. If you decide to join us I'm afraid you'll have to take part in the drill. Sit there for now and we'll have a talk later.'

Sergeant Paragon was not pleased. He had lost the first round. The second began shortly afterwards and from then on it was open warfare.

After a short talk from me the men were usually set tasks in groups of four, one of whom became the patient. Tonight there was a change.

'Alright Randall,' said Paragon, 'you lie down 'ere. You'm the patient. Everyone round 'ere. All together tonight. You four treat un ver vractured vemur, you four ver fractured skull, you lot ver vractured left radius and you ver dislocated right shoulder. Get on wi' it.'

In ten minutes Albert Randall looked like a huge doll dressed in bandages. It was difficult not to laugh and an occasional grin from the men was the least one could expect. But Paragon was not satisfied yet.

'Now a bit of artificial respiration. Schafer's method. You virst Tom.'

This meant heaving the trussed and splinted body of Randall over on to his face and at last he began to resist. I decided the initiation had gone far enough. 'Wait a minute,' I said. 'Are you suggesting, Sergeant Paragon, that your men would treat all these fractures while the patient was not breathing and set about artificial respiration last?'

'No zir, just ver practice, that be all.'

'Practice must resemble reality, I've told you that many times. If you needed to do artificial respiration you'd do that first, of course.'

''E's only just stopped breathing,' said Paragon, determined to win the argument.

'As a result of all your ministrations?' I couldn't help asking.

Paragon took this for permission to carry on. He was no whit abashed. 'Alright men. Turn 'im over. Schafer's method.'

'What is going to happen to his dislocated shoulder and all those fractures while you do that?' I asked.

'Won't do un no good, Darcter,' replied one of the men seriously.

'No, it won't. So what are you going to do?'

'Sylvester's method,' said Paragon. 'On 'is back.'

'And how are you going to raise his arms with those injuries?'

'You couldn't,' admitted someone.

'What then?' I asked.

After several minutes during which the patient might have died, someone suggested the mouth to mouth method.

'Who's going to do that?' I asked. 'Will you oblige, Paragon?'

'Not me zir.'

The voice of one of the divisional humorists came from the back of the group. 'Now if twer a noice young woman, we'd all be wantin' to 'arve a go.'

'Haven't you got a piece of apparatus you could blow through?' I asked them. 'What about the triangular mouthpiece from the oxygen-giving set?'

There was a rush to fetch it and Alby spoke at last.

'Reckon if Oi'd 'ard all thic clobber on me, Oi'd be glard to stop breathin' and get out of it.'

'Alright,' I laughed. 'Undo all those splints and bandages and let someone else be the patient.' There seemed no need to get involved in actual mouth to mouth respiration, so I suggested a change of exercise.

'Right men, get to it,' shouted Paragon. 'Charlie you be the patient now. Pressure points. Bleedin' vrom left vemoral region. The thoigh if yer don't understand the prarper wurd.'

This however was not a night noted for its smooth running. One of the men gripped Charlie firmly round the upper thigh with his thumbs superimposed on the midpoint of the groin.

There was a roar from Charlie. ''Old on,' — the verb was singularly inappropriate — 'you'm squeezin' me balls. Ruined ver bloody loife. Let go, can't yer.'

Charlie was released and a more careful effort made to block his femoral artery.

'Oi've often wondered, Darcter. Suppose twer a woman.' The speaker was one of the members not over-endowed with intelligence. 'Would we 'ave to get 'old on 'er loike thart?'

'Of course,' I said. 'You couldn't let her bleed to death with arterial haemorrhage, could you?'

'Easier wi' a woman,' said someone in a stage whisper. 'No balls to git in the way.'

'That'll do,' thundered Paragon, glad to assert himself again. And the class went on with its exercises.

Albert Randall, now properly dressed again, watched in silence. I talked to him later.

'What made you want to join the Brigade?' I asked him. 'You felt you ought to learn some first aid?'

'Oi zuppose zo, zir. 'Twer young Len Parsons did put Oi up to it. Er zaid everyone ought to be able to zave loives loike. 'Twas after thic day you stopped 'is bleedin and put 'is shoulder back.'

I told him I was due to start a course of lectures again in a few weeks and he had better start then. He needed the lectures first and the practical exercises later. Meanwhile I meant to have a word with Sergeant Paragon. It would be a pity if Randall were put off by Paragon's nagging. I need not have worried.

I told Paragon not to indulge in any buffoonery, especially with a new member. He apologised but there was no denying the undercurrent of hostility.

Randall listened carefully to all my lectures and did something I had never seen any of the others do. He took notes and I was surprised at the speed of his writing. The first time this happened Paragon said to him after the lecture, 'What were you writin', Randall, love letters?'

'I bain't zo clever as you be, Harry. Oi loike to zee un wrote down.' And somehow his broad grin seemed to establish his superiority and independence. Paragon gradually stopped his bullying.

Randall soon came to use his great hands with remarkable deftness and passed his first annual exam with top marks.

Sometimes when a man is bitten by the 'bug' of first aid he becomes as obsessed as the passionate golfer with the recognition of his efficiency. This happened to Albert Randall. He turned out to be highly intelligent and soon knew the handbook by heart, but the more he came to know about first aid the more energy Paragon spent in belittling him. Randall put up with the criticism with infinite patience, but his confidence could hardly be expected to flourish under such a barrage of hostility.

Fortunately an opportunity occurred eventually to give him a boost. I had been called to see an accident at the colliery first aid centre. It was one of the fine new buildings erected after nationalisation. While I was dealing with the case another casualty was brought up from underground. This was an unusual one. A man had been yawning and had dislocated his jaw — a remarkable thing to happen in those circumstances — and Randall had come up with him. Paragon was already in the room, having come up with the first casualty.

First aiders are not normally allowed to make any attempt to reduce dislocations, but I thought this was an exception. 'I'm a bit busy, Randall,' I said. 'Will you deal

164

with the dislocated jaw? Wash your hands carefully. You know what to do.'

Paragon was up in arms at once. 'Shall I do it zir?'

'No, it's Randall's case. He'll do it.'

It was a simple matter to reduce the dislocation and Randall stood behind the patient, put his thumbs behind the lower back teeth and pressed the lower jaw firmly downwards. The jaw sprang back into place and Randall was, I thought, surprised at his success. He showed no excitement and put a bandage on the man's face to prevent him opening his mouth for an hour or so.

Paragon looked annoyed so I said tactfully, 'You've taught him very well, Sergeant. Nothing wrong with that treatment.'

I had occasion to visit Mrs Randall some time later and she spoke of the dislocated jaw. 'Alby was main pleased wi' what you let him do,' she said. 'He'm a changed man. I never saw him so pleased with himself.'

'He's a great worker,' I told her. 'I don't know anyone else who could do two jobs as well as he does and find time for first aid as well.'

'He's always been good with his hands,' she said, 'and with the animals, but he always wanted to do something better — more skilful. He reads a lot too, you know, sir. I often think if he'd had a good education he'd have done wonderful things for himself.'

'Like a lot of us,' I told her, 'he was born too soon.'

And this was true. Twenty years later Randall's son had not only won a scholarship to Cambridge but had remained there to do research work. The younger generation of the nineteen eighties has great privileges; the whole of society has the advantage of being able to draw on the resources of gifted people who in the past would have had no chance of taking on high responsibility.

The twentieth century has not been all bad.

14

The receptionist in what used to be called the surgery but is now dignified by the more appropriate name of Health Centre is arguably the most important member of the staff — perhaps not more valuable than the doctors themselves but vitally important. This has now been recognised by the provision of special training, but even in these enlightened days a receptionist's errors of judgement may have tragic consequences.

When some sensitive soul has been debating for days whether or not the queer pain in his chest is due to indigestion he may suddenly, one Friday morning, make up his mind to phone the Health Centre and ask to see the doctor.

'Could I have an appointment with Dr X please?'

'He's very busy. Is it urgent?'

'Well not really, I suppose.'

'I could give you an appointment for next week. Would Tuesday morning do?'

'Well I'm working you see.'

'Wednesday evening?'

'I was really hoping to see him sooner.'

'If you are working I take it it's not urgent. Will you tell me what the trouble is?'

'It's nothing much. A bit of indigestion I expect.'

The receptionist doesn't realise how desperately he wants it to be indigestion and nothing worse. 'Very well, we'll say Wednesday evening the 16th at 6.15.'

When the sensitive soul dies of his coronary thrombosis on the Friday night no one knows that he tried to get an appointment with his doctor, or that the receptionist lacked the ear of experience. She merely remarks the following Wednesday evening — the day of the funeral actually —'That man didn't turn up and never bothered to cancel his appointment. Aren't they hopelessly inconsiderate, these people?'

Of course it all depends on the point of view. The receptionist had seen the harassed G.P. looking tired and pale after his last consultation. A garrulous and complaining lady had kept him far longer than necessary so the receptionist generalised her resentment against all and sundry.

If the conversation at the first contact with the receptionist had gone like this, things might have been different.

'I was really hoping to see him sooner.'

'Will you tell me what the trouble is?'

'It's nothing much. A bit of indigestion I expect.'

'Is it something new?'

'Yes, I've only had it the last week or two.'

'What sort of indigestion is it?'

'It's like wind but it isn't wind really. Keeps coming and going in the front of my chest.'

'And it worries you badly?'

'It does rather.'

'I'll give you a short appointment for this evening. Then the doctor will be able to decide.'

We were lucky with Annabel Jamieson. She had had no special training except that of a dispenser but she had good sense and a sound instinct. One morning at the end of the winter of 1950 I had some dozen new calls to do. I already had a heavy list of visits — my records show that I did twenty-eight visits that day — and I must have shown my resentment at so much work. One of the calls was to a Mr Patrick Ryddenwood who was said to be sleeping badly. In the state I was in that morning a request to visit someone because they were not sleeping well was an outrage beyond human endurance.

'Did you really have to take a message from that man? Why can't he come to the surgery?'

Annabel's colour rose sharply under any criticism but she said stoutly, 'I think he really is in trouble.'

'I don't see why his sleeping badly means he can't come to the surgery.'

'He really didn't sound well enough.'

I knew it was no good arguing. If Annabel had decided the man needed a visit he probably did.

The case stays in my memory for two reasons. First, it showed the importance of knowing a whole family when one member of it becomes a patient. The second reason was the Jekyll and Hyde behaviour of the daughter of the household.

I put the Ryddenwood visit low on my list of priorities and got to the house at about three thirty in the afternoon. New visits had to be done before four o'clock surgery, otherwise they would be too late to catch the chemist before he closed.

Patrick Ryddenwood and his wife sat one on each side of the fireplace looking thoroughly dejected. The house seemed uncared for, dusty, dark and slightly smelly. The man apologised for sending for me and went on, 'I can't stand these headaches. I've had them for days now. My head throbs and aches and sometimes I can't see.'

I was not familiar with so-called cluster migraine at that time, but his loss of vision was typical of the early stage of migraine. It would last for twenty minutes or so and would be followed by severe headache and occasional vomiting. After a few hours the eye trouble would herald yet another attack.

While I was examining him his wife was walking restlessly to and fro, picking things up and putting them down again, poking the fire, sitting down for a moment and then getting up again. I began to think that if I had to watch a wife behaving in this way I should soon be a casualty myself.

'What about you, Mrs Ryddenwood,' I asked, 'are you alright?'

'Yes, I'm alright.'

'She's not very well Doctor. She doesn't sleep properly. She wakes up at four in the morning and doesn't go off again. Then she's tired all day.'

'What about your daughter?' I hadn't seen her for a

168

year or two but she must have been old enough to take some responsibility. 'If you are both unwell couldn't she stay at home from work to help?'

'She's not well herself,' Ryddenwood answered. 'She says she's coming to see you.'

'He thinks more of her than he does of me,' put in Mrs Ryddenwood.

'That's not true, Doctor. I think the world of my wife.'

By that time in my life I had decided that the translation of 'I think the world of my wife' was 'I am sick and tired of my wife but I daren't say so.'

It was clear that the whole household was involved. The man had to be treated for his migraine, and the wife seemed depressed, while the daughter who might be helping at home had some trouble of her own.

I talked for some minutes to Ryddenwood and it became clear that his migraine was very severe indeed. I ordered him treatment then talked to his wife. She listened to what I had to say but made no reply that I can remember. She seemed depressed and may have needed treatment, but she hadn't asked to see me, so I left them saying I would discuss things with them again when I had seen their daughter. One thing was certain, Annabel Jamieson had been right and the visit had been necessary.

Selena Ryddenwood came to see me on the next Saturday morning. She was eighteen and buxom. Her lips were covered with too much lipstick, her finger-nails were painted a bright scarlet and the amount of eye-shadow she wore made her appear to be looking through a pair of black goggles. One had the feeling that with a good scrub and less make-up she would be a very attractive girl.

'I feel sick,' she said, 'and I can't eat anything.'

She didn't look ill and had no pain but she just didn't feel well. Her period was two weeks late but this had happened before. I wondered why she had come — perhaps to put in a claim to illness which would excuse her from any obligation to help her parents.

I examined her abdomen and found nothing. The possibility of pregnancy occurred to me — perhaps because of her tartish appearance — so while examining her chest I looked carefully at her breasts. There was nothing to suggest a pregnancy.

Then she asked a blunt question. 'Am I going to have a baby?'

'No, I don't think so. Do you think you might be?'

'I could be, I suppose.'

At one time a possible way of getting a favourite boy friend to marry a girl was to become pregnant by him. This thought crossed my mind and I said, 'You don't want to be pregnant, do you?'

'I wouldn't mind,' she replied and her blasé manner began to irritate me.

'Are you thinking of getting married?'

'Not unless I'm pregnant.'

'You would marry if you were?'

'I expect so.' She appeared supremely self-satisfied, shrugging her shoulders in complete indifference.

The question seemed important so I asked Annabel Jamieson to come into my room while I did a pelvic examination. It was immediately obvious that the girl was a virgin so I didn't proceed but I was more puzzled than before. The fear of pregnancy after a kiss or a cuddle would indicate a degree of innocence that was rare even in 1950. So what was the object of her visit? There appeared to be nothing the matter with her and her cheerful truculent manner denied any great discomfort.

I told her firmly that she was not pregnant but she showed no reaction and said nothing. 'You are not relieved then?' I asked.

'Why should I be? I don't mind one way or the other. It's the thing these days, isn't it? If you get caught you get married, if you don't get caught you don't get married.'

I was half horrified and half amused. This was 1950, some time before the new 'morality' became traditional. 'I wouldn't have thought that was the only reason for getting married,' I said.

'You're a bit old-fashioned, aren't you?'

This seemed about enough insolence from a teenager and I came straight to the point. The chance, I thought, that a girl like this would stay at home to look after her parents was remote, but I had to make the suggestion.

'Your parents are both really ill,' I told her and to my surprise she registered astonishment.

'Mother and Father really ill? Mother is a bit miserable and Father gets bad headaches, that's all, isn't it?'

'No, it's by no means all.' I told her what I thought about them and was aware that I was exaggerating somewhat, but it seemed justifiable. 'Could you stay at home for a while to help them out? I think if you stayed home for a week your father would improve fairly quickly.'

The girl began to look worried and I found the sudden change of expression curiously pathetic. 'How do you really feel?' I asked her.

'Not too bad. I wondered if I was pregnant, that's all.'

'You're not,' I repeated, 'and don't get pregnant at present because your parents are in trouble and need you.'

I knew I was being harsh with her but then to my surprise she said, 'Alright, I'll stay at home next week.'

At that moment she seemed to change quite suddenly from a tart wondering if she was pregnant to a responsive dutiful daughter. Her speech and her whole manner changed. The defiant half-mocking expression disappeared as at the wand of a magician, and an anxious young woman was peering out from behind the make-up. I found the experience quite moving.

I gave her a note for her employer stating the domestic situation and the immediate problem of the Ryddenwood family was solved.

I wanted to ponder the small miracle I had witnessed, but there was no time in the middle of surgery to guess at the reason for her earlier behaviour. She had clearly been acting a part for some reason of her own.

The difference in her was even more obvious when I visited the family a few days later. The whole household had changed. There was a sparkle about the place. Patrick Ryddenwood was better and spoke of returning to work shortly, but Mrs Ryddenwood was not so well. She sat silently huddled up by the fire and my concern for her grew.

'You're not feeling well, Mrs Ryddenwood,' I said.

171

Her husband replied for her. 'No she's not, Doctor. She can't sleep and she's too tired to do anything. I don't know what's the matter with her. Perhaps she needs a tonic.'

'I think I'd better have a proper look at you,' I told her. 'Go up to your bedroom and get into bed, will you?'

'I'm alright,' she said almost inaudibly.

'Go on Mother. Do as the doctor says.' He sounded thoroughly irritated by her. 'Come on, I'll help you.' And with the aid of considerable force he got her upstairs and into bed.

While I was waiting for her to undress I spoke to Selena. 'What do you make of your mother?'

'I can't understand her,' Selena said. 'She hardly talks to us. She won't go out, won't talk to the neighbours, hardly eats anything and Father says she doesn't sleep either. It's as though she was terribly worried about something.'

'Does she say she's worried about anything?'

'No, she keeps saying she's alright and just wants to be left alone. She's always a bit quiet but never like this.'

'Does she cook? Do any housework?'

'She does a bit but she's so slow. It takes her twice as long to do the slightest thing.'

Although Mrs Ryddenwood was sallow-faced and rather thin I found nothing physically wrong with her, but the combination of early waking, slowness and melancholy made the diagnosis of endogenous depression fairly obvious. What was more, she was getting rapidly worse.

Drug treatment and psychotherapy for depression were less well established then than they became later, and the most commonly used treatment was electric convulsion therapy.

I had been called to see Patrick Ryddenwood but it was now clear that the real patient was his wife. Some cases of depression worry you straight away because of the danger of suicide. I felt uneasy about this case and suggested an appointment with a psychiatrist at the mental hospital ten miles away.

Father and daughter were alarmed at the suggestion but I managed to persuade them that it was necessary.

I was still puzzled about Selena's strange behaviour in the surgery earlier and as she walked out with me to my car I said, 'I'm glad you've taken a week off work to help at home.'

'Well it's my job, isn't it? The trouble is there's not much money coming into the house. Only Father's sick pay and that's not much.'

'I was puzzled by your visit to the surgery the other day. You weren't really worried about pregnancy, were you?'

'Not worried, no.'

'You knew you weren't, didn't you?'

She laughed evasively. 'A bit daft of me really, I suppose.' And I got no further enlightenment.

I think Mrs Ryddenwood's appointment with the psychiatrist was made for a week later, but it was before six o'clock in the morning a day or two later that a very worried Selena telephoned me.

'It's Mother, Doctor. She's gone out somewhere and we don't know where she can be.'

'You mean she's not in the house or garden?'

'No, I can't think what's happened to her.'

'Can I speak to your father?'

She was ringing from a call-box and it would take five minutes to get him so I changed my mind. 'How long has she been gone?' I asked.

'About half an hour, we think. Father thought she had gone downstairs to make a cup of tea but when he came down ten minutes ago she hadn't even put the kettle on. If she went straight out when when she got up from bed she would have been gone about half an hour.'

Half an hour. And I had a terrible feeling I knew where she had gone. 'I will come over,' I told Selena, 'but I'll drive round the lanes and have a look for her on the way.'

The Ryddenwoods lived about two and a half miles from a place called Emboro Pond. This was a fair-sized lake, very deep and surrounded by trees. It was a dark and lonely place, and during my twenty years in Melbrook at least two people had committed suicide by drowning themselves in the lake. Mrs Ryddenwood had been gone half an hour and it would take little longer than that to walk to Emboro Pond.

I dressed more quickly than I had done for a long time. 'What is it?' Jessica asked me.

'You know that Ryddenwood woman I've been worrying about with depression, she's gone off this morning after not leaving the house for days. I've got a horrible feeling she's making for Emboro Pond.'

'Oh how awful. Do be careful.'

In a few minutes I was driving as fast as I could towards Emboro. I decided it was best to make straight for the 'pond' and, if there was no sign of her there, to make my way back towards the Ryddenwoods' house in the hope of cutting her off. As I drove along the Wells road I tried to think of any other plausible reason for the woman going off without warning before daylight. I could find none. The worst time in the depressive's day is the early morning when life can be almost intolerable. This is consequently the commonest time for attempts at suicide. With every minute that passed I was more weighed down by the thought of what I was going to find. If Selena's assessment of the time factor was accurate her mother would reach Emboro just before I did.

I raced along the main road to the point where she would have joined it, then strained my eyes to see to the limit of the beam of my headlights. There was no one on the road except one cyclist. For a moment I thought of stopping to ask if he had seen anyone on the road, but decided it wouldn't help if he had.

I drove on, my heart pounding against a leaden weight in my chest. I turned left into the lane that bordered the pond, then swung the car round so that its headlights shone along the length of the water. And there she was, standing by the water's edge.

If she jumped in now, how in heaven's name was I going to get her out? Jumping into that icy water with my clothes on to try and drag out a woman determined to drown herself was a very grim prospect indeed.

I got out of the car, leaving the headlights on, and ran

towards her. I had no plan other than to grab hold of her. Then I remembered that other woman before the war who had thrown herself out of her bedroom window on the Mendips, and I was afraid I might frighten her into precipitate action. I called after her as calmly as I could and walked towards her. She was standing absolutely still, a yard or so from the water's edge, so I got between her and the water and said with exaggerated calm, 'Let me take you home, Mrs Ryddenwood. You must be half-frozen.'

To my enormous relief she made no opposition and allowed me to lead her back to the car. I still had the worry that she would leap out while we were going along. We had no seat belts in those days and there was no way of controlling her. I half decided to stop at one of the cottages in Emboro village and ask for help, but this would mean a lot of publicity for the poor woman and anyway she seemed almost unnaturally calm by this time.

So we drove home to her house and I put her in the charge of her husband and daughter while I phoned the mental hospital for an emergency bed. She was admitted that day and made a full recovery in about three months. In her case the electric convulsion therapy worked very well.

I was left wondering what would have been the outcome of the case if I hadn't been called to see the husband for his migraine. How soon would they have sent for help for the wife, and would the call to say she had left home early one morning have been the first intimation that she was ill? If so, there would have been nothing to make me undertake a mad chase after her and arrive just in time.

Of course it was possible that she never intended to jump into the water and would have gone home on her own, but I didn't think so.

Annabel Jamieson had made a shrewd decision that morning when she told me the man who couldn't sleep needed a visit. I asked her how she had made up her mind and she said, 'Oh I don't know, it was the way he talked. I felt sure there must be something really wrong there.'

'Clever girl,' I said.

If one member of a family is ill, then as often as not the

whole family can do with a little unobtrusive help. Sometimes the one really causing the trouble is hidden in the background.

By this time I was intrigued by the whole Ryddenwood family, particularly by the strange behaviour of the girl when she first visited me in the surgery. I talked to Jessica about her that evening. It had been a traumatic start to the day and it always helped if we could mull over difficult or puzzling cases together. I had of course already described in detail the affair at Emboro Pond.

'That girl Selena,' I said, 'she's really a very nice girl, obviously kind-hearted and fond of her parents. The change in that household when she took over was extraordinary. You know how one good caring personality can affect a home. Yet it was the same girl who came to the surgery painted up like a prize tart, asking whether she was pregnant when she knew jolly well that she was still a virgin. I can't believe it is the same girl. She evidently likes to act the part of a promiscuous woman of the world when she isn't. But why? A proper Jekyll and Hyde.'

It was a domestic scene in our old study at The Elms. We always used that room when we were alone. It had a red brick fireplace with bookshelves to the ceiling on each side, and my desk by the window. We had our deep armchairs one on each side of the fire and spent some of our happiest times there.

Jessica didn't answer for a moment but went on with her sewing — probably repairing torn garments belonging to the younger two girls. Then she asked suddenly, 'Do you remember that man Gaynor?'

'Archibald Gaynor? Yes, why?'

'Don't you remember how puzzled you were about him at one time? You talked about a Jekyll and Hyde personality then. He came to see you one day and had become a completely different person.'

'Yes, I remember.' And my mind went back to an interview before the war that is still vivid in my memory.

Archibald Gaynor was a scholarly man of great dignity and solid personality. He must have been in his late forties, unmarried, successful and quite well-off. He always ran expensive and exotic sports cars but otherwise he was a model of sobriety, active in charitable works and committees. He seldom consulted me but I knew him well. He was slim and fit and took great care of his health.

That was the man I knew, or thought I knew, quite well until one day he came to see me in his other personality. As soon as he came into my surgery consulting-room I sensed the difference. He asked after my health and seemed rather full of himself — as though he had just made some remarkably astute deal on the stock exchange.

It took several minutes of unusual sparring before he came to the point and then he said casually, 'I'm afraid I've picked up a dose of clap.'

One is startled often enough in a lifetime in general practice but for a moment I was shocked into silence. Not by the disease, but by the disease in this man. If the Archbishop of Canterbury had come to me boasting that he had just succeeded in robbing the Bank of England I should have been no more astonished.

'Gonorrhoea?' I managed to say rather lamely.

'Yes, came on yesterday. May I have some treatment?'

I examined him, took the necessary tests and started him on treatment, then referred him to a consultant. Gonorrhoea was much less easy to treat before penicillin, but sulphonamide was available by then so there was a good prospect of a cure. Before sulphonamide a single dose of gonorrhoea might be followed by a lifetime of strictures, suspicion and misery.

In due course the condition cleared up and the tests were satisfactory. He came to see me for a final chat and then it was that I was truly shaken by him. There was no embarrassment or regret. His manner could only be described as blasé — or perhaps cocky would be a better word. He seemed quite proud of himself.

'All clear now,' he said, 'so when can I have a woman again?'

Keeping my professional mask as firmly in place as I could, I replied, 'It depends on the woman. Not the one who gave you this?'

He laughed happily. 'Oh no, I shan't see her again. I

177

shall choose more carefully from now on, I can assure you.'

'I think you are safe now not to pass on any infection,' I told him.

'Never condemn your patients in your manner or in your mind' is a very good precept. This time it was difficult to carry out. We parted friends but with some chilliness on my part, I fear.

'I wonder what's happened to him,' I said to Jessica. 'I haven't seen him or even thought about him since the war.'

'Didn't I tell you? He committed suicide during the war while you were away. It was rather horrible. He got into trouble with some small boy and — well — couldn't face the disgrace I suppose. He shot himself.'

'Good heavens!' Then light dawned on me in a flash. 'So *that* was it. He was a homosexual all the time. All that talk of going with prostitutes was just a facade. Poor devil. He was trying to prove to himself and the world that he was normal — or what we call normal — heterosexual I mean. What a pathetic story. Poor, poor devil. Why haven't you told me before?'

'I don't know. It was a long time ago and all rather horrible. Perhaps I tried to forget it.'

'But it's not horrible, it's tragic. The poor chap was fighting to be "normal", to prove he was not a homosexual. How he must have loathed the thought of going to a prostitute again. I'm sure he didn't intend to, but he pretended he would when even the thought must have made him want to be sick. That of course accounts for his extraordinary behaviour.'

We sat for a time in silence. Jessica's mind always shied away from perversion or sexual abnormality of any kind. To her, sex and love were synonymous. One without the other was unthinkable.

I went on pondering the case. It still stays in my mind as one of particularly poignant sadness. If only I had realised his problem and could have discussed it with him freely, his life might have been very different. I had dismissed him with chilly prudery when I ought to have been searching for an explanation of his behaviour.

Presently I said to Jessica, 'What made you tell me about Gaynor now?'

'You were telling me about the Ryddenwood girl, and when you said Jekyll and Hyde it reminded me of how puzzled you were over the Gaynor case.'

'Oh I see.' And again my mind raced away. 'This girl couldn't be a lesbian trying to prove she is not one, could she?' I asked.

'I've no idea.' She concentrated on her sewing and we dropped the subject, but I was still puzzled. Jessica had probably worked the Gaynor problem out in her own mind and had come to the same conclusion as I had, but didn't want to talk about it. Hence her suggestion that the Ryddenwood case might be a parallel one.

It must have been a couple of weeks later that I had a phone call from the cottage hospital one Saturday evening. There had been a brawl in the High Street and a youth had been cut on the head. Bleeding was difficult to control so I was sent for to do some repair work. As far as I remember there was no trouble over stopping the bleeding except that the boy was terrified as soon as he saw the suture needle. As so often happens, young men who go about in gangs and are full of aggression become simpering wrecks as soon as they are confronted by the threat of pain in strange surroundings. I detest violence and the show of aggression and am not good at giving these young men a sympathetic understanding.

'What did you do to make the other lad attack you?' I asked.

'Just told 'un to get back to Bristol where er belonged.'

A few stitches under local anaesthetic soon had him in fairly good shape and he began to swagger immediately he got off the operating table. 'How many stitches?' he asked.

'Not enough to boast about,' I told him.

When I left the casualty theatre the boy's companions — two girls and another boy — were sitting waiting for him. Both girls were heavily made up and I went by without taking much notice. After I had passed them it suddenly struck me that one of the girls' faces was familiar, so I turned to look at her. It was Selena Ryddenwood — not the pleasant girl who had been looking after her parents, but the other Selena, the one who had consulted me a week or two ago in the surgery asking if she was pregnant. She was made up in exactly the same way with scarlet finger-nails, painted face and black goggle eye-shadow.

'Are you alright, Selena?' I asked her.

'I'm O.K. The boys were having a bit of a shindy, that's all.'

'You'll have to keep him out of mischief, won't you?'

'It wasn't him. The guy from Bristol just set on him.'

'Oh Selena,' the other girl protested.

'He didn't mean it — what he said.' She was defiant, brittle. This was Selena Mark Two alright.

I suddenly felt sure that she was no lesbian and an idea which had probably been lurking at the back of my mind came to the surface. 'May I have a word with you?' I said. 'I want to talk to you about your mother.'

I walked along the corridor with her and asked how her mother was getting on.

'She's O.K.,' Selena said and she spoke as though she couldn't care less but the tone was obviously unnatural, affected.

'You mean she's better? She was terribly distressed when she left for hospital, you remember.'

Then I watched her expression change before my eyes. Hyde was becoming Jekyll again.

'She had that treatment,' she said, 'that electric treatment. She seemed a bit better.'

'I expect it will help, but it will take time. What about your father? How are you managing at home?'

'He wanted me to stay at home from work and run the house but I didn't want to.'

'You ran things so well before that I thought you enjoyed it.'

'Mother was at home then.'

'Any special reason why you don't want to stay at home now?'

180

She hesitated. 'I don't know. I think it's better for me to be at work.'

'I've been wondering whether there was any special reason for your mother's depression. You haven't any idea yourself, have you?'

'I don't think Mother and Father get on very well together but they've always been like that.'

I couldn't ask any more direct questions so I concluded the conversation. I was just leaving her when she said, 'Father had one of his migraine attacks again yesterday.'

'Is he worried about your mother, do you think?'

'No, not now. I think it came on because I wouldn't stay at home from work.'

'Tell him to come and see me if he gets any more.' So I was left, still wondering, but with a few more clues to the puzzle. Her parents didn't get on well together, that was one thing, and she was happy to stay at home when her mother was there, but not alone with her father.

There was probably some degree of parallel with the case of Archibald Gaynor, but if she was not a lesbian what was she running away from? My guess was that she and her father had had a close emotional relationship. Her projected image of herself as a promiscuous woman of the world might be her way of escaping from a threatening relationship with her father.

All this was only guesswork, of course, and part of my continued effort to understand people — especially the strange ways of teenagers. I may have been completely wrong, though I don't think I was, and anyway my theory was better than condemning the girl for behaving like a tart.

Patrick Ryddenwood and his wife settled down to a 'normal' life after her recovery, but I thought the strong attachment between father and daughter might well have been at the root of the wife's depression. The great battlefield of family life is responsible for many casualties. The only thing the doctor can do to help is to try to understand the pressures and emotions that beset every family where the parents have not had the good fortune of a strong lasting mutual attraction.

Selena made a successful marriage in due course and I watched her children grow up in a good secure home. Most problems solve themselves if one can only wait long enough.

15

Looking over Jessica's postwar diaries, I am amazed at
the extent of her activities. There is a constant stream of
entries. 'So-and-so came to stay; had the — children for a
week while parents were away; gave a talk to —, felt very
nervous.' One of her most heroic activities was her habit
of making regular visits to Miss Crabtree. This great country character lived in a cottage near our first home in
Melbrook — so near, in fact, that it became inevitable that
Jessica should send her in a Sunday dinner each week and
generally keep an eye on her. But Miss Crabtree was no
ordinary old lady.

An honest description of her is likely to be thought pure
fabrication, but I will tell the truth as I remember it. Her
clothes must have been in the height of fashion in the
eighteen nineties and would have been still acceptable at
the turn of the century. Her black dresses were ankle-
length with leg of mutton sleeves, tight waist and skirts full
enough to take a bustle. I think her single concession to
modernity had been the removal of the bustle. Her black
boots shone brilliantly and on rare occasions revealed
their elastic sides before disappearing under the volumi-
nous folds of her skirts. Her grey hair was always neatly
coiled on the top of her head and only once in thirty years
did I see a hair out of place.

Apart from some dental deficiency, she was very good-
looking, had regular features, a slim elegant figure and the
posture of a guardsman standing before his commanding
officer. Her skin was as clear as that of a healthy young
woman and her blue eyes had a constant challenge which
seemed to say 'Now, now, what have you been up to? I

don't believe you anyway.' Her words were chosen and spoken with great care and an obvious effort to eliminate the slightest trace of the Somerset accent we so dearly loved. She was, I think, of gentle birth but her 'gentility' when we knew her was somewhat exaggerated.

She was the owner of the Cedars, the house we rented from her for the first five years of our life in Melbrook, and it was of the utmost importance to her that her tenants should be what she termed 'professional people'. A popular surgeon in our firm had lived there until his death in 1918 but later she had been obliged, she told us, to lower her standards and had let the house to a pleasant couple she had regarded as positively lower middle-class. Being a doctor I apparently passed her test and we were welcomed in 1930 as though she had been waiting for us for years. Jessica, of course, won her heart in about five minutes and never lost her adoration.

She was my patient for some twenty years without ever a thought of consulting me. In fact she made it politely clear that she had no personal use for doctors.

'It's my belief, Mrs Lane,' she said to Jessica one day, 'that if people took proper care of themselves there would be no need for doctors. Nothing personal of course. My father,' the words were spoken reverently, 'my father never had a doctor until the day before he died at the age of eighty-one. Yes. . . .' And there was more than a hint that had he avoided the medical profession then he would have been alive today.

In 1935 we had moved to a house large enough to accommodate our increased family but Jessica still kept in touch with Miss Crabtree. I saw little of her but had accounts of her increasing eccentricity from time to time — an eccentricity which showed itself by the number of cats that shared her cottage. Very occasionally I was asked to give advice on questions like the 'outrageous' nature of rates demands or the threats of robbery with violence from the inspector of taxes, otherwise I was not consulted. It is well-nigh impossible to keep twenty odd cats in a small cottage without producing a powerful smell, but this was where Jessica's heroism showed itself. Her visits remained regular.

One day in the late summer of 1950 a child brought a note at breakfast time asking me to call on Miss Crabtree. There was no mention of trouble with the legal profession or the collectors of rates or taxes, but that she had suffered from a pain in the chest for two days and would be glad of something to relieve it.

I announced my amazement over the breakfast table. What had happened? We had thought the stars would stagger in their courses before she would send for a doctor. A chest pain in someone who not only never asked for help but didn't believe in doctors was something to take notice of, so I decided to visit her before surgery. The wording of the note might have warned me that what was expected was a magic pill which would cure without delay or inconvenience, but if so I took no heed of the warning. I walked into the lions' den that morning almost blithely, because I was glad she had changed her mind about seeking medical help.

I was received at the door by the lady herself and was struck at once by two things — first by the smell of cats that escaped from the cottage as soon as the door was opened, and second by the fact that it was clear that Miss Crabtree was not at all well. The contrast between her elegance of manner and the pale lined face was quite remarkable.

She was wearing a black cape over her dress in spite of the warmth of the day, she had lost her colour and her face was lined with strain. It was so obvious that she was really ill that I didn't even experience my normal desire to stop breathing for the duration of my stay in such an unsalubrious atmosphere. I would normally start breathing again when my olfactory sense had been reduced by fatigue and at the same time my body had developed a violent need for air.

On this occasion I was immediately concerned with the business in hand, and my first inclination was to get her sitting or lying down while I examined her. 'Will you lie on the couch, Miss Crabtree,' I said to her.

'Certainly not, Doctor. I am not as bad as that. I will sit here if you wish. Please to sit down yourself.'

'Tell me about the pain in your chest,' I asked.

'It's nothing serious. I'm sorry to have to trouble you.' Her breath was short and suggested a chest infection. 'If you would be so kind — as to give me something for the pain — I should be most grateful.'

Against considerable resistance I managed to extract a history of her illness. Two days before, she had had a shivering attack and felt as though she was catching a cold. The pain came on soon afterwards and was increased by deep breathing. Then she began to sweat and feel constantly chilly. She couldn't eat anything and had been unable to sleep for two nights. I couldn't help admiring the courage of someone living alone who was prepared to face a second night of severe pain without asking for help. I expected to find a blatant pleurisy or perhaps a patch of pneumonia — enough to force ninety-nine people out of a hundred to bed and an early call for help. A brief examination should clinch the diagnosis and I could order treatment to begin at once.

'Slip your dress over your shoulders, will you,' I said, 'then we can decide what to do to help you.'

She made no move but sat bolt upright, looking at me with more than her usual challenge.

'I shall have to examine your chest,' I repeated, glancing at my watch which told me I ought by now to be in the surgery.

'Doctor Lane,' she said, 'did I hear you say take my dress off? Did I hear aright?'

'Yes, that's right.'

She rose with some difficulty and drew herself up to her full height, her breath coming a little faster than before. Then she spoke in her most royal manner. 'That I can't agree to do under any circumstances. Never in my life have I exposed myself to a man.'

'But I'm a doctor, Miss Crabtree,' I said. 'I don't understand. I can't treat you unless I find out what is the matter.'

'I think Doctor knows very well what is the matter. I've got pleurisy. That's what it is, pleurisy. So I need some medicine.'

Never in my life — and I had been qualified for twenty-two years — had I treated pleurisy or anything like it without examining the patient, and quite suddenly I became as stubborn as she was. She might be suffering from shingles for all I knew. The situation was ridiculous.

'I can't tell the cause of the pain without examining you, Miss Crabtree. Please undo your dress so that I can make a proper diagnosis.'

She stared at me, her hands clasped on her lap. Then her manner changed and she began to wheedle. 'I think Doctor has already made his diagnosis. And I think Doctor is clever enough to give me something to stop the pain. I know he is.'

'I'm sorry. There's nothing I can do without an examination.'

'Then I'm sorry I troubled you, Doctor. I must wish you a very good morning.'

'I shan't have a very good morning unless I find out what is the matter with you and get you on to some proper treatment. Why don't you want me to examine you?'

'Because you are a gentleman, Doctor. And I am a lady. That is the reason.'

So what was I to do? I couldn't leave her without treatment and I couldn't force the clothes off her. Then a thought occurred to me. The district nurses — Martha and Mary — lived opposite her cottage. They would help, of course.

'I'll go and get the nurses,' I said. 'You will allow them to undress you, and I can examine you while they are here.'

'No.' The word was violent. 'I don't like them. I won't have them in the house. Common women. No, I shall manage on my own. I'm sorry to have troubled you.'

By now I was quite touched. I found the courage of this dear old lady, living all alone, battling through two nights of severe pain very moving. Her quaint ideas must have been indoctrinated by strange Victorian parents and her excellent health had prevented the need for examination for many years.

I considered the possibilities. I could refuse to give

treatment without examination. This might mean leaving her to get worse and perhaps to die. I could give treatment without making a proper diagnosis. The ideal treatment, if she had a patch of pneumonia, was penicillin, but at that time this could only be satisfactorily given by injection and it was certain she would refuse to undress for this. I could admit defeat and give her sulphonamide tablets, hoping for the best — or — I could get help. Tom Wyburn would meet with the same refusal to undress, and I knew he would not treat her without examination. There was only one person who would be likely to handle this situation successfully, and that was Jessica. She had been a nurse at Guy's but more than that, she would know better than I did how to handle Miss Crabtree. I could pick her up after surgery and we would do the call together. All I could do meanwhile was to give a couple of veganins with a drink of milk from the kitchen. This would aford some temporary relief.

'I shall be back after surgery,' I told her, 'and I shall bring Mrs Lane with me.'

'Yes, I would like to see Mrs Lane. I'd like to see her very much.'

I always went home for mid-morning coffee after surgery and Jessica was usually there to greet me. Looking back, I realise how much I took her care for granted. I can boast that I was nearly always punctual for meals unless some emergency intervened, when I would telephone the house. This is only a matter of sensible organisation and people who fail to take the trouble to get home in time for meals are usually either lazy, muddled or selfish. I am often all three, but not over this particular problem of general practice. In return, my meals were always ready and I was able to eat at once and often be out again in fifteen or twenty minutes. I was sometimes accused of resembling a vacuum cleaner, drawing in the food and moving on again. Not a very flattering description of a sociable occasion, but the work was heavy for ten years after the war. Mid-morning coffee, on the other hand, was at variable times according to the length of the surgery, and if I was late she might be out. That day I was lucky and was able to explain my problem of the undressing of Miss Crabtree over coffee.

'What happens if she refuses to let me undress her?' Jessica asked.

'I shall put her on sulphonamide and hope for the best, but I feel I ought to make some serious effort to examine the old dear.'

When we arrived at the cottage I realised that giving veganin had been a tactical error, adding considerably to my difficulty.

'I'm much better, Doctor. The tablets have done me a lot of good. I was sure it was just a matter of the right medicine. A few more of those and I shall be quite alright. Oh Mrs Lane, so good of you to come.'

Jessica had brought an egg custard which was to have been for the children. Beth and Catharine both attended Miss Thatcher's school and came home to lunch. 'I'll leave this for you,' she said and looked at me for guidance.

'Miss Crabtree,' I said, 'you may have pleurisy, and that means I shall have to give you some strong tablets. But I can't do that unless I know what the trouble is, so I *must* examine you.'

'But all I want is some more of the same tablets. I don't need anything stronger.' She smiled as though the matter was amicably settled.

Jessica indicated that I should leave her with the patient, which I was only too pleased to do. This sort of ridiculous situation could quickly become infuriating on a busy day. I took a turn in the little garden, wondering how things would go. In about two minutes I went back inside only to find Miss Crabtree sitting in her chair fully dressed. I thought perhaps I had been a bit too quick so I went to the window and looked out. Jessica was talking non-stop. 'What a horrid thing to have. You must have had two dreadful nights. Why didn't you send for me before? If it's pleurisy it's serious but the doctors can cure it now.' And so on and so on. Meanwhile she was unbuttoning the old lady's dress and in a short time her chest was exposed for examination.

In five minutes I had examined her with no trouble at

all. She had a patch of pneumonia and fairly extensive pleurisy on one side with a temperature of a hundred and one — probably reduced by the veganin.

She was in her sixties and would be better off in hospital. This meant the Royal United or St Martin's in Bath, either of which I felt sure would take her. Now that I — or rather Jessica — had won the first battle I thought she would cooperate, but far from it. Even Jessica was powerless to persuade her. If she went to hospital she would die. This she knew. She would not leave her cottage for anyone.

I promised to look in later in the day, then left a prescription with a neighbour who agreed to get the sulphonamide from the chemist. Penicillin was still very expensive and was not at that time used as extensively as it was a year or two later.

As we left the cottage I said to Jessica, 'How did you make her so amenable? She didn't utter a sound when you undressed her.'

'I don't think you'd be very flattered,' she laughed.

'Go on, tell me.'

'I told her that doctors are neither men nor women, they're just doctors, and this seemed somehow to console her.'

'You little devil,' I said, 'you of all people should know me better than that.'

Miss Crabtree made a fairly rapid recovery. I didn't do battle again to make a further examination in spite of the image I had been given as a non-man. She was not ill again for some fifteen years.

The interesting postscript to the story is that she had an attack of bronchopneumonia when she was approaching eighty. This time I insisted on her being admitted to the cottage hospital which was by then taking medical cases.

'I shall die if you send me to hospital, Doctor. I know it. I shall die.'

'This time I insist,' I said.

She died some four hours after being admitted to hospital.

16

Farmer Lyle was a successful man but always seemed to be carrying a great load of trouble he never talked about. He was friendly, good-humoured and easy to talk, yet for several years I had no idea what was tormenting him — until one day in September 1933.

His wife was a quiet woman, not one who would ever be regarded as the life and soul of the party but a model of the efficient farmer's wife. Jonathan, the son, aged twenty-five, was very much a man of Somerset, well built, blue-eyed and with a voice that could be gentle or dictatorial according to his mood. He and his younger sister Anna were a complete contrast to their parents. Anna was a gentle soul, her Somerset accent as soft and warm as a feather bed. Their main characteristic seemed to be an inborn happiness, they were always cheerful, teasing and jolly. To a geneticist the contrast between parents and offspring might have represented quite a remarkable phenomenon — until, that is, the family secret became general knowledge.

I was called to see Farmer Lyle one Saturday afternoon in September 1933. He had taken to his bed with acute lumbago. The pain came on suddenly and all but immobilised him. The treatment we gave for lumbago at that time was identical with that used when the cause of the condition had later been identified as disk trouble — rest on a firm bed and relief of pain, followed by care to avoid heavy lifting and the use of a supporting belt if necessary.

When I had dealt with him, I met Jonathan and Anna downstairs with a young woman who appeared to be a friend of both. They were having tea and, being offered a cup, I accepted it. There were no inhibitions about the younger Lyles and Jonathan was talking in his usual clear voice — probably audible some half a mile away. 'Now young Meg,' I remember him saying, 'you'm a farmer's daughter, what would you do if one of your best cows slipped her calf?'

The girl named Meg was solidly built and obviously of equally solid character. She replied without hesitation. 'If 'tis only one, do nothing but if it happens again, get the vet and find out whether you've got fever in the herd.'

'That's what I'm worrying about. This is the second case. Well Mother, you heard what Meg said. It'll have to be the vet. I shan't worry Father. He's got enough to think about at the moment.'

'It's going to cost you a bit if he wants to test them all.' Meg was evidently a practical young woman who already had a considerable interest in the Lyles' cattle. Her eyes were all for Jonathan and his for her. It was pretty evident from their manner that there was romance in the air.

Mrs Lyle was dispensing tea and large slabs of bread and butter, cream and jam in the farm kitchen, a room some twenty feet square with a huge fireplace at one end now occupied by an Aga cooker. She seemed restless and kept leaving the table to go to some other part of the kitchen. When she came back to her place at the table she was still fidgety, which wasn't like her. The thought passed through my mind that perhaps she was worrying unduly about her husband so I talked to her about him, saying that in a couple of weeks he would probably be about again but would have to leave any heavy lifting to Jonathan and the other men. She took little notice of what I said and suddenly I noticed that the fingers of one hand, as well as her face, were making small spasmodic movements. Facial spasm is a very common condition and very embarrassing, and I supposed this was the cause of her being ill at ease. Shortly afterwards I took my leave and it was only with hindsight that the tea party came to have any special significance.

I visited Farmer Lyle twice more and after the third visit Anna followed me out to my car. 'I wanted to have a word with you about Mother,' she said. 'I can't make her out. She's getting so forgetful and bad-tempered and she's so fidgety. Someone said they thought she had St Vitus' Dance, whatever that is. Have you noticed her twitching? I thought I saw you looking at her that first time you came to see Father. I felt sure you'd noticed it but you didn't say anything.'

'Yes, I did notice it, but what did you mean about being forgetful? Is she worried about something?'

'I don't know but the other day she went to Melbrook shopping. She had a big list of things to get and she came back without half of them. Then when I told her about it she got quite nasty. I'm wondering what's the matter with her.'

I am not sure at what stage the true diagnosis occurred to me, but looking back it seems as though I suspected it from that moment. St Vitus' Dance — chorea — choreiform movements with evidence of mental changes, the earliest of which could be forgetfulness. Am I flattering myself or did the truth occur to me straight away? I don't know.

'I think I'd better have a look at her,' I said.

'She'll be furious if she thinks I've said anything.'

'If you are worried you must make her see me.'

'She'll never come down to the surgery. Are you coming to visit Father again?'

'I wasn't planning to. I'd better come back and see her now.'

'She won't like it. I shall get it, mind.'

I led the way back to the farmhouse and confronted Mrs Lyle. 'Anna thinks you are not well, Mrs Lyle,' I said. 'You aren't feeling well, are you? And you are getting these twitchings in your face.'

'Oh that's nothing. Anna's no business to have said anything. Just a bit run down with Father being ill, that's all 'tis.'

'Can I have a look at you?'

'No you can't. What should I want to be examined for? I'm perfectly alright I tell you.' Her colour rose and she was clearly getting very upset. 'You're a stupid girl,

Anna.' The words were spoken with real venom. She was evidently ill but there was little I could do about it unless she cooperated.

'Alright Mrs Lyle,' I said. 'But if you think I can help you must let me know.'

I retreated and Anna followed me again. This time she sounded nervous. 'There's something else, Doctor. I ought to have told you. I was talking to Father about it. He told me there's something in the family. It's a sort of insanity.' She held her breath for a moment. 'I don't know why he never mentioned it before, but now he says an older sister of Mother's went insane when she was thirty and died when she was about forty. And it's possible my grandfather — Mother's father — may have had it, but he was killed in an accident and they were never sure. Isn't it awful?'

'Yes, it sounds worrying. As soon as your father is well enough you must get him to insist on your mother seeing me.'

I left feeling very unhappy indeed. The family history of insanity added to my suspicions that the condition I was faced with was Huntington's chorea. I looked it up as soon as I got home. It is a rare hereditary disease which shows itself by choreiform movements together with mental degeneration and this proceeds to complete mental and physical breakdown over some ten to fifteen years. The worst thing about it is that it has a dominant inheritance, which means that each child of an affected parent has a fifty-fifty chance of inheriting it. If Mrs Lyle had Huntington's chorea both Jonathan and Anna — those delightful people — had an even chance of developing it. If they did inherit it, their children would have an even chance of inheriting it too. On the other hand, if they escaped it their children would be perfectly safe.

The evil thing about this disease is its way of dicing with something far worse than death. According to which way the dice falls, the individual at risk is either doomed to develop it or is completely free from it. Equally distressing is the fact that it may strike its victim at any age from twenty to seventy. The result is that those with an affected parent will spend their lives not knowing whether or when they will contract one of the worst diseases known to man. And their children will be watching them with desperate anxiety, because if they do develop it the next generation will be at risk too. If they do not, their children will be free, untainted and healthy.

It is hard to imagine a worse cat and mouse situation than the one arising from Huntington's chorea. My mind rebelled against it. Was it possible that a good God had ordained that this disgusting disease should toy with the lives and happiness of human beings in such a way that they would never know, from one day to the next, whether they would die a miserable death of utter degeneration of mind and body, far worse and more long drawn-out than any cancer? And the chance of developing the disease is not just one in twenty, like that of a heavy smoker who might develop cancer of the lung, but even chances.

I had been qualified for five years, but I couldn't remember a harder assignment than explaining the full horror of this condition to Jonathan and Anna Lyle.

That evening I was thoroughly depressed. I couldn't even talk to Jessica about it at first, and after dinner I sat staring into space. A vile disease is bad enough if you meet it in a complete stranger, but in someone you know and like it is much worse. The dread of it would, if possible, be worse than the reality, and the years of anxiety that Farmer Lyle had been through must have been a torment. I seemed to see the evil shadow stalking him over the years until it finally caught up with him.

I came back to reality as I had done on a few occasions in the past, aware that Jessica was sitting on the arm of my chair, her hand in my hair. 'Aren't you going to tell me about it?' she asked.

As always her closeness stirred me to life. 'It's the most bloody thing I've ever come across,' I said and told her the whole story. 'Suppose in April 1927 we'd discovered that my father had Huntington's chorea, what should we have done?'

'We'd have married but had no children,' she said.

'Are you sure? No children when you could have

195

married any one of a dozen healthy young men?'

'Of course I'm sure.'

As far as our feelings for each other were concerned there never were any problems, but no children — this would have been a bitter disappointment. Apart from a lifetime of anxiety. I tried to imagine myself heroically going off to some foreign land and leaving her to make a new life with someone else, but I knew very well I shouldn't have done it.

In due course I examined Mrs Lyle and sent her to see a neurologist who confirmed the diagnosis. At the same time I wrote to the British Medical Association library for literature about the disease. I wanted to construct a graph to show the percentage risk at different ages for the members of an afflicted family. As always, the librarian gave me a degree of help that I have long wanted to pay tribute to. I received a series of articles about the disease, including some with accounts of families in America which had suffered from it.

When I had mastered all the facts I could find, I arranged to talk to Jonathan and Anna in the surgery one Sunday morning. This was the best time for any long discussion, when the chance of interruption was least. And so it came about that I faced them in my room in the old surgery on a Sunday morning in November 1933.

The most urgent problem was that of Jonathan's intentions to the girl named Meg whom I had met briefly at the farm. I began by facing this head on, without showing any of the sympathy I had been feeling. It would have been all too easy to get bogged down in a morass of despondency which wouldn't help either of them.

'Knowing that your mother has got Huntington's chorea,' I said, 'your risk of getting it, assessed at birth, was exactly fifty-fifty. But ten percent of the people who have it develop it in their twenties, so this means that by the time you are thirty your risk will be that much less. In fact it would be forty-five percent. Every year after that your risk would be less, until by the time you were sixty the chances would be down to five percent if you were still free from it. And by that time the risk for your children would be half your own risk — two and a half percent. And you know that if you don't inherit it they will be absolutely safe from it. There is no question of any sudden throwback in later generations. Once you know you don't carry the disease your descendants are safe.'

They were an intelligent couple and had naturally been thinking a lot about the problem of their future, so they understood what I told them very quickly.

'I'm twenty-five,' said Jonathan, 'so in five years I shall still have a forty-five percent chance of getting it. We've been saying fifty, but forty-five isn't much better.'

'And I'm twenty so my chance is still fifty percent,' Anna said.

'Are either of you thinking of getting married?'

'Well I'd been thinking about it,' Jonathan replied. 'You saw young Meg over at ours?'

'Yes. Have you made any plans?'

'She's made up her mind about it. She's broken it off — what there was to break off.'

'I'm sorry.'

'I'm not. If that's the way she wants it, let her go, that's what I say.' He was doing his best to show his independence, but I knew him well enough to understand by his manner that he was deeply hurt.

'And you, Anna?'

'I'm not thinking of marrying anyone and never shall. That's definite.'

'There's nothing to stop you marrying and having no children,' I told Jonathan.

'That wouldn't suit Meg. She's out for her own good and no one else's.'

'You can't blame her, Jon,' put in Anna. 'You'd be the same, so would I.'

'I'm sorry about your girl, Jonathan,' I said, 'but it does mean you've no decisions to make at present. If either of you ever do want to get married you could plan to have no children and that would reduce your worries and responsibilities, wouldn't it?'

'You've got to find someone willing to marry you,' remarked Anna, laughing for the first time.

'That may very well happen,' I said. 'After all, you are a very attractive girl and there is a fifty-fifty chance that you will be as healthy as anyone else and will live till you are ninety. A good many men would be happy to take the risk.'

It suddenly struck me that the chance that either Jonathan or Anna would develop the disease was almost a hundred percent, but there was no point in saying so.

'What I can't understand is why neither Mother nor Father said a word about it long ago. They knew what was in the family but kept it to themselves.'

'We knew that Mother's sister died young,' Anna said, 'but not that it was anything hereditary.'

'I don't see any point in your parents telling you about it. There was nothing you could do about it except worry. And for all they knew your mother might never have developed it. Then there would have been nothing to worry about.'

'Suppose I'd got wed and started Meg in the family way before Mother got ill?' Jonathan said.

There was no answer to this, except perhaps this was what they had intended, but I well understood how the parents had pushed the whole matter on one side in the hope all would be well. We talked all round the subject for some time and they seemed to feel a little better for giving it a good airing.

The solution to their problem came slowly and what impressed me most was the attachment that grew between them.

The first time I realised the closeness of the relationship between brother and sister was in 1938. I met Anna in the town and she was radiant. 'I'm going to be married,' she told me.

I was delighted. I didn't know the young man she was to marry but was sure she would make a good choice. 'I shall have to come and see you about you know what,' she said. Birth control was not such a matter of routine knowledge from the age of ten onwards as it is now and I guessed what she meant. It was a joy to see her so happy in spite of the family disease.

It must have been several weeks later that she came to see me in the surgery and she was not looking at all happy then.

'Is it about birth control?' I asked.

'No, it's not really settled yet. I've been miserable. It's Jon, you see. He's perfectly sweet about it but he's taking it awfully badly. Anyway why I came to see you was that I can't sleep. I go to bed and just lie there. It's awful. I just lie there all night worrying about poor old Jon.' She looked at me wide-eyed, as though no one had ever suffered from insomnia before.

We talked about her engagement and about Jonathan for a while and then I said, 'This is an occasion when you have got to put yourself first. Jonathan will miss you but your marriage comes before anything.'

'It's not so easy as that. You see I'm very fond of Jon. There's no one really like him. I feel different about Billy — my fiancé — of course. He excites me. It's wonderful. Yet every time we get close together alone I seem to see Jon's sad face looking at me.'

'You'll have to put your feelings for Jonathan on one side,' I told her. 'Your marriage is far more important. You shouldn't hesitate. Jonathan will recover once you are married and as likely as not he'll marry too.'

'Do you really think so?'

'My advice is to put yourself first. It's not natural to let a brother stand in the way of marriage.'

We talked for a while and she left with some sleeping tablets and a promise that she would take my advice.

But of course she didn't.

Some weeks later Jonathan came to see me. This was the only time he consulted me about himself in twenty years. It was a matter of headaches. And of course the cause of the tension was Anna's impending marriage. I did my best to persuade him that it was a great blessing that his sister was to marry. 'She'll have a far more satisfying life than if she remained single,' I told him. 'Do you like the man?'

'Oh, he's alright. An ordinary sort of chap and he doesn't care about children. He just wants Anna and I don't wonder. She's as pretty as a picture.'

'Once she's married you'll accept the situation,' I said, 'and be glad for her sake.' I gave him something for his headaches and told him he must make things as easy for Anna as possible.

The affection of brother and sister for each other was understandable enough because thay had so much in common, but it had to be kept in perspective.

He left me, girding himself to face the inevitable, and I congratulated myself on giving the right advice.

The next thing I heard was that Anna's engagement had been broken off.

The war came and then for four years I saw nothing of them. During that time their mother had to be committed to a mental hospital and their father died. My next encounter with them was very different. By this time they were both in their thirties and living together in perfect harmony.

It was, I think, the first Bath and West Show after the war. It happened to be a fine day — a rarity for the Bath and West — and Jessica and I were wandering round the grounds when we ran into the Lyles. I hadn't had occasion to see them since I came out of the army and it was quite a reunion. We talked together, the four of us, for some time and then Jonathan dragged me off to see some machinery he was keen about.

A little while later we saw Jessica and Anna Lyle talking and laughing together like old friends as they strolled in the sunshine.

'Look at those two,' said Jonathan proudly. 'As like as two peas in a pod. What a lovely couple!'

Jessica said to me afterwards, 'What a sweet person Anna Lyle is. There's something about her — personality, mystique, or whatever you like to call it. And she seems perfectly happy living with her brother.'

'She was engaged to be married before I went away but she broke it off. I suppose she couldn't bear to leave her brother. Amazing, isn't it?'

'She's terribly fond of him.'

'And he of her. But I can't understand the relationship being so close.'

'I can.'

'A life without sex?'

'I think they could have an almost sexual love without sex if you know what I mean.'

'No, I don't.' This was beyond me at the time.

What impressed me most was that the usual family grouping of husband, wife and children was not the only way to a satisfying life. I learnt through them that a brother and sister relationship can be very profound. I suppose the sexual instinct is sublimated into a degree of companionship that can only be described as intense. When it is encountered — and I have only met it once in my life — it is a moving experience.

Neither Jonathan nor Anna ever married but they lived together very happily. Their love for each other became obvious over the years. Anna grew into a most attractive woman, slender, lithe, with an almost transparently lovely skin and a personality that combined strength with a touch of magic and mystery. Her appearance convinced me that she was happy.

I never brought up the family disease but when Anna was about fifty she spoke about it herself. 'I'm sure neither Jon nor me will get the family trouble,' she said. 'I feel somehow that we are alright.'

As one who believes strongly in the feminine instinct I was delighted to hear what she said. Incidentally she was probably right. I have to say 'probably' because it was not long after that that she developed a cancer.

I watched Jonathan go through the shock, the false hopes and the final despair you would expect from a devoted husband. When she had been discharged from hospital after an exploratory operation he took personal charge of the nursing through the many weary months that followed.

Anna would sit in their sun-room placidly reading or looking out over the fields, and one day she said to me, 'The only thing I can't bear is the thought of leaving Jon to live alone. I can't bear to leave him.' And she wept bitterly for a moment until she regained control.

Just before Christmas 1963 I admitted her to the cottage

hospital for terminal care but still Jonathan spent nearly all his time sitting beside her. By that time we had learnt a good deal about the relief of pain in cancer, and it was usually possible to ensure an easy and even comfortable death. The relationship that then sometimes develops between doctor and patient is unique.

I said to Jessica one evening, 'I think in a strange sort of way I'm a bit in love with Anna Lyle.'

She looked at me quizzically, waiting for me to go on. 'It's an odd thing, but you get extraordinarily close to people sometimes when you both know they are about to die. You've been through months of illness together, battled through the pain together, shared so much — I can't explain it.'

Later that night she was quiet, withdrawn. 'What is it?' I asked her. 'What's the matter?'

'I think I'm a bit jealous of Anna Lyle,' she said.

'How can you be?' I laughed. 'It's not that sort of love.'

'I should be an awful wife if you were the sort of man who ran after other women.'

'Well I'm not that sort. And neither, thank God, are you.'

Anna's life was clearly drawing to a close and Jessica and I had long planned to go up to our doctor daughter's home in Chester for Christmas. I knew I should have to leave Anna to die in other hands and I told her I was going away for three days When I paid my last visit to her before we left she said to me 'I shan't see you again then, Doctor. Thank you so very much for all you've done. I could never thank you enough.'

For I think the first time in my professional life I had to struggle to hide the tears that welled up into my eyes. I stood holding her hand, ostensibly feeling her pulse, for more than a minute, then I forced a smile and said 'Goodbye, Anna' and left her.

When I came back after Christmas she had died and Jonathan was heartbroken. He had hidden his grief for months but at last it had to burst into expression. I shall never forget his tears as he sobbed over and over again, 'What am I gonner do without her? What am I gonner *do*?'

202

He lived several years after her death but never developed Huntington's chorea. They might both have married and had children if they had acted according to the instincts of nature without any thoughts for the future. Even so, I don't believe they would have been any happier.

A deep love for another human being is the one thing — for many of us the only thing — that makes life worthwhile. It is all too rare, even between husband and wife. I believe it occurs occasionally between two men and in this case it certainly existed between brother and sister.

Men of religion are apt to look askance at what they call 'inordinate affections'. I believe they are wrong. Real love between two people is always good. It can bring glimpses of heaven into a sad world and should be sought after like a holy grail. This love Jonathan and Anna shared in full measure and no one should ask for more.

17

I have saved one quite dramatic story almost to the end of this volume. It serves to illustrate the importance of giving patients the opportunity to know the truth about themselves, and it highlights the tragedies that could occur if they are kept in ignorance of the real state of their health.

It concerns a man named Austin Crisp. He was one of those men who seemed to have everything, looks, money, health and a cheerful disposition. He usually dominated every conversation he was involved in. When I met him socially it was interesting to watch other men, who were also dominating extroverts, gradually give way to him until he became the centre of attention. He was a social being and loved to entertain. I knew him fairly well during his first marriage — a happy one with an only daughter. Sarah, the daughter, was a very pleasant girl but the opposite to her father in character — quiet, shy and rather a dreamer.

In due course Sarah was married and soon afterwards her mother was killed in a road accident. Poor Austin was shattered — utterly desolated. For a year the life seemed to have gone completely out of him. He lived alone with daily help in the house, smoked incessantly and drank a lot. Some of his friends tried to keep him company but soon gave up the effort. As is often the case with men of his type, he had virtually no close friends. Being popular and a natural entertainer had given him all he needed in life — so long as he had his wife.

It must have been about two years after his wife died that I heard he was being seen about the city with an attractive young woman. He was about fifty at that time and she was reported to be in her early thirties. She was a stranger to the area — Austin lived some miles out of Melbrook — and I supposed she was either a widow or divorced. Everyone who knew Austin was delighted and it became an accepted thing that he would remarry. There seemed no point in delay and when there was no marriage after a year his associates were surprised. I didn't know anything about the young woman and imagined, if I thought about it at all, that she had to wait for a divorce to be granted her. Later another possible and very different explanation occurred to me.

In due course they were married and Austin resumed some of his old sociable habits. When I met the new wife for the first time, he seemed head over heels in love with her and she was certainly an attractive woman. With Austin's money she dressed well and their home became a showpiece of good taste. Many things in the house became a focus of envy among the women of the nearby city — those, that is, to whom things mattered more than people. I attended Austin but we did not meet them socially.

All went well for several years until, when Austin was about sixty, he came to see me one evening complaining that he had been coughing up blood. He made very light of it and said he had only come because Helen, his wife, insisted that he should.

'Strained myself, that's all. This smoker's cough in the morning, you know.'

I couldn't find any signs in his chest and had difficulty in persuading him that an Xray was necessary. This was done in the city hospital but gave us no more information. I recommended him to see a chest specialist who I felt sure would suggest bronchoscopy — a direct examination of the bronchial tubes — but he absolutely refused. Only when he had further haemorrhages two months later could he be persuaded to see a consultant. This was done in Bristol and a cancer of the lung was found.

At that time operation was less commonly attempted and he was given radiotherapy only. I expected him to come home from the chest unit depressed and deflated, but he was perfectly cheerful. They had been guarded in what they said and he had assumed there was nothing seriously wrong. His wife, on the other hand, was told the truth.

'All a lot of nonsense,' he told me. 'And you wouldn't believe me, would you?'

After a couple of months he decided to 'take a rest from work'. He ran a large business but had good managers and this was quite easy to do. As the weeks went by he seemed to be losing ground but had little or no pain. He became somewhat breathless and lost weight so I thought it was high time he should realise what the trouble was. Usually in such cases one feels one's way carefully and the opportunity comes when the patient asks why he is not improving, but Austin never asked a single direct question. He was still remarkably cheerful and took everything as it came.

When he began to get chest pain I felt I really must have a straight talk with him. He was still planning extensions to his business when he got better, which didn't seem fair on him or his business or his employees. I discussed the matter with his wife first. 'I don't think he can last many months,' I said to her, 'and he ought to be told he can't get better so that he can make any plans he thinks are necessary.'

'No, he mustn't be told,' she said. 'He could never face it. We should be torturing him. I'm so glad he's been able to persuade himself that he will get better. Surely you'd rather let him die peacefully without knowing what's going to happen.'

'He's bound to know sooner or later,' I said.

'Then let's wait till he guesses,' she answered.

'Do they know at the business that he won't come back?'

'I haven't told them, but I think they do.'

'I think they ought to know. Have you talked to your solicitor about that?'

'No, I haven't in fact.'

'Do talk to him. He really ought to know what is happening.'

She was silent for a moment. 'I'm so afraid he'll find out. You see I keep telling him he's getting on well, and if he finds out from someone else it will look bad for me.'

I wasn't at all happy about leaving him in ignorance, but I supposed that when he felt worse he would demand the truth from me. Sometimes patients know very well what is wrong but can't face talking to other people about it. Perhaps he knew more than he admitted and had already put his affairs in order.

When he began to need drugs to relieve pain I decided I ought to take further advice, so I telephoned his solicitor whom unfortunately I didn't know.

'I'm not asking you to betray any confidences,' I said to him, 'only to advise me whether I am right or wrong in letting Austin Crisp believe he is going to get better.'

'When he won't?' he asked.

'Yes. Helen, his wife, is determined that we should go on letting him think he will recover as long as possible, for the sake of his peace of mind. Are his affairs in order?'

'His business affairs are in order, yes.'

'Right, but you know how difficult these things can be. I thought as his solicitor you ought to know the true state of affairs — in strict confidence of course. Then if there is anything he ought to do, you would be able to advise him.'

'I'm grateful to you. I had heard rumours but I'm glad to know about it.'

After that I decided I had done everything possible, and was prepared to let him think for a time that he would recover. Then I happened to meet Sarah, his daughter, when she was visiting him one day. She had run into serious trouble since I had last seen her and had developed rheumatoid arthritis. As I was leaving the house she said 'Could I come and see you — not about myself — about Father I mean?'

'When are you going home?' I asked her. 'Would you like to come down to the surgery this afternoon before you go back to Bath?'

This was arranged and I met her there at about two o'clock.

'I think I ought to tell you straight away that Helen and

I are not the best of friends,' she said. 'What worries me is that she has assured Father that he's going to get better when he obviously isn't. I don't want to sound terribly mercenary and I wouldn't have said anything except that I'm in desperate trouble. My husband has left me and he's being terribly difficult about money. So far I have refused to divorce him. Even if I do and if I got all the courts allowed me, I should still be very badly off. And you see I can't go to work because of this wretched arthritis. Well, what I'm coming to is that when Father married he changed his will. He told me that as I was quite well off — or my husband was — he had left all his money to Helen. I think — I can only think she insisted on this before she would marry him.'

'And you mean that if he knew he was going to die he would make some provision for you?'

'I'm certain he would. He said the other day that as soon as he felt better he was going to put things right for me.'

I told her that I had already alerted his solicitor and it seemed up to him to make sure Austin's will expressed what he intended.

'But do you think it's right that Father is being told lies about his future?'

'No I don't. It's always safer if people are told the truth. Helen, of course, insists that if he knew his case is hopeless it would only increase his suffering — which may be true. Leave it to me. Somehow I'll make sure he knows the truth.'

Next day I visited Austin and told his wife before I saw him that I must insist on his knowing what was really wrong with him. To my surprise she didn't argue. I had suspected her of not wanting him to change his will and keeping him in ignorance of his real state because of this, but perhaps I was wrong.

Then I had a session with Austin. I was much younger then and I hated it. I still do, of course, but perhaps the misery is forgotten more easily than it used to be.

He was silent and shocked. I had thought he might have had his suspicions, but he hadn't. 'Helen told me it was an

208

inflammation of the lung and it would clear up in time but I had to be patient.'

'Didn't they tell you in hospital what it was?'

He shook his head in puzzlement. 'No. All they said was that I should feel worse for a time after the Xray treatment and then I should feel better. I didn't cross-examine them.'

I felt very sorry for him. He seemed to shrivel before my eyes and clearly Helen had been right to some extent. By taking away all hope I had increased his suffering. I tried to mitigate things by saying there was 'never a never' in medicine, and cancer did sometimes regress, but at the same time he would have to be prepared for the worst and put his affairs — both family and business — in order. He didn't say anything about what he must do, he was too overwhelmed by the sudden change in his outlook.

After that I waited, hoping sooner or later to hear something about a new will, but nothing happened.

As I watched him deteriorate over the next few weeks I wondered whether I had been right. I talked to Tom Wyburn about it and he said — probably correctly — that my only duty had been to let the solicitor know that he would not recover. Apart from that, his wife had a perfect right to try to keep him happy by telling him he would get better.

I doubted my action more as the days passed, and my uncertainty made me talk the affair over with my old friend and ex-partner Edward Evans, who was then practising in Bath. He said at once, 'He ought to be made to make another will.'

'You can't do that, but surely his solicitor ought to make sure he is satisfied with his will.'

'I'll tell you why I said that, Ken. There have been rumours that Helen Crisp is seeing a good deal of Sarah's husband.'

'Good heavens!' I was shocked. Edward Evans was always well informed about Bath gossip and I didn't doubt what he said. This put an entirely new outlook on the whole business. It was possible to suspect the most dire of intrigues. Was Helen going to inherit all Crisp's money and then link up with Sarah's husband? And would she use her power over the money to force Sarah to divorce her husband? I couldn't really believe this but it was possible. On the other hand, for all I knew Sarah and her husband might have made things up and he was only seeing Helen to put Sarah's point of view about a new will.

When I thought things over I felt more and more uneasy. Even the kindly Sarah had admitted she didn't like Helen, and suspected that she had insisted on a change in Austin's will before she would marry him. This fitted in with the unexpected delay in their marriage.

There was only one thing I could do. I must get in touch with Austin's solicitor. This was a Sunday and we were having lunch with Cicely and Edward Evans as we often did. I phoned the solicitor the next day and asked if he had seen Austin recently.

'I can't seem to get hold of him,' he said. 'I've telephoned twice and was told he was not well enough to be seen. Then I called there the other day and he was so doped that it was impossible to get him to listen to me. I agree with you but I'm afraid we've left things rather late.'

I then suggested a plan with which he concurred.

Day and night nurses were in attendance on Austin by that time because regular doses of morphia were needed to relieve the pain. I told the day nurse that the dose of morphia the next morning was to be drastically reduced. Then I calculated when the pain would become more severe and went to the house at that time. The solicitor had agreed to be there at the same time.

The pain was increasing and I had the dose of morphia made ready. 'Before I give you the injection,' I said, 'is there anything else you want to do? Your solicitor has just called and if you want to talk to him we could have him in before I give it to you.'

The pain in his chest made him catch his breath and seemed to put everything else out of his mind. 'Business affairs?' I asked. 'Family affairs? Will? Your mind is quite settled about family matters? Sarah struggled along to see you again yesterday, didn't she?'

At last it came. 'Wait a minute,' he said. 'I haven't

made that will. I told Helen to get Bertie along. I haven't done it, have I?' Bertie was what he called his solicitor.

I sighed with relief as the solicitor came into the room and within a short time the new will was made while he was clear in his mind. I was called back to witness his signature and then gave him his dose of morphia.

And were my suspicious of Helen completely unfounded? So far as any intrigue with Sarah's husband was concerned, they were. She was left comfortably off and wasn't married again for some years and then not to Sarah's ex-husband. I was glad of this because it left me free to consider her innocent. All her actions, when one came to think of them afterwards, were compatible with a desire to keep her husband free from worry. Except perhaps — but I don't know.

The whole point of this story is that if a patient doesn't know he is going to die, all sorts of unfair things can happen. In this case, by the time Austin Crisp knew the truth he was needing drugs for the pain, so he neglected to take action that would normally have been automatic.

As things turned out, Sarah was well provided for and all ended as well as it could. All the same every patient has a right to know what is happening to him when he is seriously ill.

18

Miles Trufitt had probably, like most of us, made many mistakes in his life but the greatest of all, it seemed, was his marriage. His wife was a woman of strong character. Had there been a competition to discover the most strong-minded woman on the lines of the Miss World contest, she would have won it hands down.

I entered the family circle once a year with monotonous regularity, on the occasion of Miles's annual attack of influenza. It would usually be in January, sometimes in the spring and occasionally in the late autumn. On Tuesday November 4th 1952 I was sent for to see him.

When she admitted me to the house Mrs Trufitt greeted me without enthusiasm. 'It's his usual,' she said. 'Feeling very sorry for himself of course.'

Mrs Trufitt was one of those women whose lower chest projects many inches forward and whose outline drops vertically downwards from that projection. In other words the lower chest, abdomen and thighs were equally prominent and no skill of corsetry could make her look anything other than a battleaxe. Her hair was mousy grey, her eyes unusually pale and her face made of corrugated india rubber. I guessed she had ruled Miles with a rod of iron for thirty years.

I offer some description of her appearance in the hope of explaining my assessment of her character.

They had an only daughter, Charlotte, who was a real charmer. It seemed typical of Mrs Trufitt that she was quite capable of defying the laws of heredity, though how a woman like her could produce a girl like Charlotte I couldn't imagine. She was lively, intelligent and friendly.

212

I followed Mrs Trufitt up the stairs, my eyes on a level with her gluteal region. This gave a clear indication of the firm pressure of corsets, which were able to confine the flesh but not by any stretch of the imagination to render it shapely.

'He kept me awake most of last night,' she said, 'demanding cough medicine, dry pyjamas after a night sweat, cups of tea, all night long. When Miles gets the flu, everyone has to know it.'

Miles was feeling miserable. He had heavy catarrh, a painful cough and a high temperature. It turned out that he had a severe attack of what could be called bronchitis, bronchiolitis, or congestion of the lungs, according to how seriously you wanted the relatives to take the patient's condition. In this case I thought Mrs Trufitt would be more inclined to nurse him carefully if I spoke of congestion of the lungs. So I did.

'It doesn't sound like pneumonia to me,' said Mrs Trufitt.

'I didn't say it was pneumonia.'

'You said he had congestion of the lungs. Doesn't that mean pneumonia?'

I don't often resort to medical jargon but I needed its help in dealing with Mrs Trufitt. 'In this case,' I said, 'it means severe infection, not of the alveolae which would be called pneumonia, but of the bronchioles — the terminal bronchial tubes — which you can call bronchiolitis if you prefer it, but which is reasonably described as congestion of the lungs.'

I ordered routine treatment together with sulphonamide tablets in the hope of controlling the infection, and promised to call again in two days time.

Late that evening I had a phone call from Mrs Trufitt. 'My husband is making a lot of fuss about feeling ill,' she said. 'Is there anything you can give him to make him sleep?'

'Has he got any pain?'

'He doesn't say so and he would certainly complain if he had. He just keeps saying he feels bad and I'm afraid he won't sleep. I told you he kept me awake most of last night.'

'Yes, you told me. Is he drinking well?'

'Yes.'

'Eating anything?'

'Some milk pudding, that's all.'

'Did he say he would like to see me?'

'No, I'm just asking for something to make him sleep.'

I ordered rho veganins to be repeated in four hours if necessary and to be taken with a warm drink.

'That means I shall have to get up at two o'clock again.'

'If necessary, yes. You sleep in another room so you could give him a bell to ring if he needs you.' I was not being unduly sympathetic.

'Can't you give me anything stronger?'

'It wouldn't be wise.'

'Very well.'

Next day I was passing the Trufitts' house and decided to look in and see how Miles was getting on. His wife was out and he was alone but no worse.

'How did you sleep?' I asked him.

'Not badly.'

'Your wife phoned last night to say you were feeling very bad in yourself. Are you any better?'

'Oh yes, I'm not too bad. I disturbed her a lot the night before and I expect she felt she could do with a better night.'

'You mean she wanted you to have a sleeping draught so that she could sleep?' I smiled at him to remove any offence from the question.

He nodded but didn't smile. He was a very serious man. 'I didn't call her last night anyway so she slept well. She needs her sleep more than most people. Feels really bad if she doesn't get her eight hours.'

I left him wondering at the way some husbands and wives stick up for each other, even when they are dealing with obvious selfishness. Was I, I wondered, too critical of Mrs Trufitt because of her manner and appearance? Anyway, if he was satisfied with her, that was what mattered. I had long ago given up asking myself why some husbands or wives gave in so completely to the other. It is sometimes because the alternative would be even more intolerable. A weak hysterical wife, for instance, may be more than a match for the strongest-minded husband. He may be incapable of understanding her, and finds that giving in to her on every occasion is the only possible way to peace. Shakespeare's *Taming of the Shrew* is a pleasant fairy tale which is not in the least like real life! At the same time he who interferes between husband and wife usually deserves the snubbing he will surely get.

It took longer than usual that year for Miles to recover, but he was back at his work in Bath after three weeks.

It was a few weeks later, on Christmas Eve, that I next had dealings with the family. When I went home for lunch Charlotte was waiting for me in their car outside the house. 'Anything wrong?' I called out to her.

I stopped my car in the entrance and she came over to me. 'It's Father, Doctor,' she said and began to laugh. 'He's been to the Greyhound and he's really very drunk.'

Miles Trufitt drunk? I couldn't believe it. He was a very precise and proper man. 'Too bad,' I said. 'But it *is* Christmas Eve. Will you be driving him home?'

'That's the point. He'll get the most awful wigging from Mother if I take him home like this. She'll never let him forget it.'

'But what can I do about it?'

'Could I bring him up here in the car for you to have a look at?'

'I shan't be able to sober him up.'

'No, but — well, if I could tell Mother he had come to see you because he wasn't feeling well. . . .'

'Then perhaps we could give him time to sober up?'

'Well, yes.'

'How bad is he?'

'He's pretty obviously drunk. Unsteady on his feet and can't talk very well. And he keeps laughing.' Charlotte laughed again at the memory. 'I've never seen him so happy.'

Poor chap, I thought, a pity I couldn't order him a small overdose of alcohol every week to cheer him up. 'Where is he now?' I asked.

'He's sitting down in a window seat with Mr Galley,

215

laughing away and really enjoying himself, bless him.'

'You'd better rescue him as soon as you can. He won't be very safe with Swain Galley. Can you manage him, do you think? No one will notice if he's a bit drunk in the pub, but once he's outside it will be more obvious and your mother is bound to hear about it.'

'I can manage him but may I bring him up here? As long as you've seen him I can tell Mother he wasn't well. And he isn't, is he?'

'Alright.' I was rather puzzled. Had Miles Trufitt really acted entirely out of character and allowed himself to get drunk? It was very unlikely. Swain might have persuaded him to drink too much but he wasn't the sort of man to be led astray by anyone. Swain's idea of a whisky, as I had discovered socially, was four-fifths of a glass full of whisky with a teaspoonful of water, but he wouldn't get that in a pub.

I went in and had my lunch. Twenty minutes later there was no sign of Charlotte or her father, so I waited. I hadn't much to do in the way of work. Everyone is too busy on their own account over Christmas to worry about doctors except in emergency.

It was easy to imagine the scene down there at the Greyhound. The pub was next to the little post office, which had already become much too small for the growing town of Melbrook, and adjoining the square which was at the heart of the place. It was a meeting ground for some of my friends.

Mervyn Davison would probably be there, the man who a few years earlier had performed the biggest act of unselfish humanity — or Christian charity, call it what you will — that I had ever known. He took into his own home a young Pole, a virtual stranger, who had developed active tuberculosis. He had nowhere to live and had to wait many months for a bed in a sanatorium. It was a year or two before the antibiotic treatment of TB was discovered; the sanatoria were full and had waiting-lists. Mervyn was young then, good-looking and quiet-voiced but shrewd. He knew very well the risk he was running. He suffered for it but recovered.

Next to him I could imagine Denys Pryce — in this case he will not, I am sure, mind my using his real name. Denys was a schoolmaster, large, jovial, intelligent and kindly. The boys at Downside called him 'Full Price' to distinguish him from a smaller colleague of the same name who was called 'Half Price'.

Next to him I could see Dr Jack Furlong sipping his pint of ale and making the others laugh by the skilful use of his mild stammer as he told his jokes. They would be country jokes about country people, well calculated to increase the sense of wellbeing on Christmas Eve.

Then I could imagine Guy Beresford, his natural tension relaxed by the pleasant company and access to a drop or two of the gin that had been in such short supply since the war.

Lastly I could see Humphrey Blaythwaite, a good doctor like his father and his brother, but at that time sorely tempted to turn his splendid voice to account and become a professional singer.

Sitting among the group I could see Swain Galley. Was he responsible for making Miles Trufitt drunk and if so, how had he done it? I seemed to have regular skirmishes with Swain over his practical jokes and sometimes suspected him without the slightest cause.

Just before two o'clock Charlotte drove up to our front door with Miles sitting placidly beside her. I went out to speak to him. 'I hear you have been having a drink with Swain Galley,' I said.

'Eshelent fellow. Shplennid commany.' Miles beamed at me and it was hard not to laugh out loud. The contrast with his usual dignity and rigid reserve was really funny. I could just imagine what his wife would have to say if he went home like that.

I told Charlotte to drive him down to the surgery and I would follow. The easiest thing for a quick cure was a stomach washout, but I didn't think he would cooperate very willingly and without adequate nursing help it would be impossible. And if I took him to the cottage hospital it would soon become common knowledge.

Just as I was leaving the house the phone rang. It was

217

Swain Galley. 'One of your patients has been indulging too much at the Greyhound,' he said. 'Miles Trufitt. Can't hold his drink. Have you seen him?'

'I suppose you knew he was coming here.'

'That pretty daughter of his told us he was being brought to see you. That was the only way she could get him out of the pub. Do you want any help?'

He wouldn't have telephoned unless he had been in some way responsible. Now he wanted to enjoy someone's discomfort, otherwise his joke would have been no fun at all. 'No thanks, Swain. I imagine you've done your part.'

'What do you mean by that?'

'How did you manage to make him drunk?'

'What bloody nonsense you do talk.' And with his usual snort he rang off.

I was more suspicious than ever now that Swain had been up to his tricks. He was capable of anything. The last I had heard of him was that he had telephoned the Bishop of Bath and Wells at five o'clock on Easter Sunday morning because the church bells were ringing early. He demanded that they should be stopped so that he could get some sleep. It suddenly struck me that if someone could gather all Swain's stories and put them in a book they might make enough money to cancel out some of the trouble he had caused.

I followed Charlotte and her father down to the surgery, led Miles into my consulting-room and made a brief examination. There was nothing more than a mild attack of alcoholic intoxication, but I couldn't let him go home like that. On the other hand, his wife might by now be worrying about his absence.

'I'll telephone your mother,' I said to Charlotte.

'What will you say?'

'I'll tell her that he's not feeling well, that I've brought him to the surgery and you'll drive him home as soon as he feels better.'

I did this and was soon facing Mrs Trufitt's cross-examination.

'Where was he taken ill and what's the matter with him?' she said.

'I understand he was in the Greyhound. Charlotte went to meet him there but he wasn't well enough to come home. I have him in the surgery at the moment with Charlotte. He's suffering from a stomach upset which I am sure is not serious. As soon as he feels better Charlotte will bring him home.'

'If it's a stomach upset, what has upset him? He won't have eaten anything since breakfast and that couldn't have done him any harm. A boiled egg and toast wouldn't hurt anyone.'

'He may have taken a snack at the Greyhound, I don't know. I'm just letting you know why he is late home for lunch. He is quite safe and will be home later.'

'If he has a stomach upset why doesn't he come home at once? I can look after him.'

'He's not feeling well enough, Mrs Trufitt.'

'I would like to speak to Charlotte please.'

I listened while Charlotte gave the same replies almost word for word to what must have been the same questions that I had been asked. In due course we both appeared to have passed the test, and like conspirators we looked at each other and burst out laughing.

'Wait here for an hour,' I said, 'and I'll be back. Then if he seems alright you can drive him home.'

In the end Charlotte took her father home at about four o'clock and as I heard no more in the next day or two I assumed all was well.

It was some time later that I ran into Mrs Trufitt again. She went into the attack at once.

'You knew what was the matter with my husband that day,' she said. 'He was drunk. That was all. He was drunk.'

'What makes you say that?'

'Swain Galley rang me up the same evening and apologised. He said he had put extra gin in Miles's drink without telling him. He didn't realise that he wasn't used to so much and might be upset.'

So my suspicions of Swain had been right, but I didn't at first realise the implications of his confession. 'He really admitted it?' I said. 'I'd suspected him from the first. I knew something must have happened because Miles would never get drunk normally.'

'And you had me worrying about food-poisoning.'

'I told you something had upset him and he would soon be alright.'

'Knowing he was drunk?'

'I admit it.'

'And why shouldn't I be allowed to know he was drunk?'

Now I was really up against it. Although I had guessed Miles was drunk through no fault of his own, my real motive had been to protect him from his wife's wrath! What was I to say now? Subterfuge was useless. 'A lie which is half a lie is ever the worst of lies' had been one of my father's strongest precepts. It had influenced me all my life. Frank admission was necessary but I didn't want to hurt her feelings.

'To be perfectly honest, Mrs Trufitt,' I said, 'I thought you would be unnecessarily ashamed of him.'

'You mean I should have been unnecessarily critical.'

I hesitated. 'Yes.'

'How little you know me.'

The conversation ended amicably but I didn't feel particularly friendly towards Swain Galley. For once in a lifetime his conscience had driven him to apologise and this had made things truly embarrassing as far as I was concerned. Typical Swain, I thought. He had come out of the affair better than I did. However the end result was not all bad.

I didn't meet Mrs Trufitt again for about a year — until Miles's next attack of flu. The advice and the medicine were more or less the same as usual, but as we were walking downstairs Mrs Trufitt said, 'It's not a stomach upset this time then?'

I was puzzled. Her expression had not changed. 'Stomach upset?' I repeated.

'Due to a snack at the Greyhound perhaps?'

Suddenly I realised she was laughing at me and I felt myself relax. 'I'm sorry about last Christmas,' I said. 'I was really acting for the best.' And I laughed.

220

For the first time in my life I felt at ease with her. Outwardly her manner never changed but mine did. And because of the change in me we got on splendidly from that day onward.

Perhaps Miles Trufitt's marriage wasn't so bad after all.

In this volume of my diary I have tried to show how I gradually learnt a little more about human nature and how I learnt not to misjudge the characters of my patients. This aim is as important as the study of the treatment of disease, as essential as is the need to keep in touch with the vast advances in medicine. What is more, the search for this illumination is more difficult than it sounds, because the personal element of the equation is variable. As the case of Mrs Trufitt showed, my own behaviour had to change before I could observe her properly. It was as though I was looking through a lens out of focus and this had to be corrected first.

When men regard themselves as stationary while the sun, moon and stars move round them, their ideas are subject to error. The same applies to the emotional reactions of the individual. The behaviour of other people varies according to our own attitudes, and we have to see ourselves as part of the problem we are trying to solve.

It is a truism to say that we are learning all our lives, but in general practice the process of learning has the advantage of continuity. You can see your mistakes. Indeed you must live with them and are likely to learn from them unless you are blind, deaf and hidebound. I want to end this volume by an example of the value of this continuity of experience. In this case it was valuable in teaching me a little more of tolerance and understanding, and I hope that on the whole it was valuable to the family concerned.

The story of Bob and Bridget Stanford is spread over many years, but one of the characters I shall mention is still alive and I have to devise a means of making the family unrecognisable. What I write may safely be regarded as true, but the facts have been rearranged so as to defy recognition and I would advise no-one to try to puzzle it out. I am trying to convey a truth which is larger than the details I write.

In the early nineteen thirties, when the problem of unemployment was even worse than in the nineteen eighties, a young man named Bob Stanford was working four days a week in the mine. For this he earned one pound forty pence a week and out of this he paid rent of thirty pence, which left him a little over a pound a week to live on and feed and clothe his wife and child. With a deficient diet it wasn't surprising that the child developed bronchopneumonia. At the same time, during the winter of 1931, Bob was laid off work.

Bronchopneumonia was almost invariably treated at home at that time, which meant that I saw a good deal of Bob during the baby's illness. In money terms he was no worse off, because five days dole was a fraction more than four days earnings, but he was acutely miserable, demoralised by feeling unwanted, and bitter over the fact that he couldn't afford the simplest necessities for his family. Bridget, his wife, had a little help from her family, but this only made him feel all the more aware of his own helplessness.

I realised then for the first time the full misery of unemployment for a vigorous man. At first he busied himself in the house trying to mend their leaking roof with pieces of wood he picked up somewhere. After a while his spirits sank steadily. He used to go for long walks by himself and come home tired and hungry to the main meal of the day, which I saw often enough that winter. It consisted of a large plate of boiled potatoes. Sometimes there would be a small rasher of fat bacon on top of the pyramid and sometimes an egg, occasionally nothing. I don't remember seeing Bridget eat. She was a splendid girl, sturdy, attractive, and reliable. Their cottage was at the end of a row, cold and damp. Conditions were grim.

The child recovered in due course and at my last visit Bob said, 'I don't want any charity. I shall pay your bill if you give me time.'

I told him that of course there would be no bill. If he had

223

any spare cash he ought to spend it on the family.

He didn't like this and replied that he would much rather pay his way.

Soft talk was no good to him and I said sharply, 'Of course you would but you can't and that's an end of it.' The hurt to his pride was the real pain.

A week or two later I was called out on a Saturday night to a girl of nineteen or twenty who was bleeding badly. Her mother thought it was a heavy period but the girl insisted that I should be sent for.

In the bedroom she somehow persuaded her mother to let her talk to me alone. 'It's not a period,' she said. 'It's a sort of injury. I went with a man this evening for the first time and it hurt me. I've been bleeding ever since.'

'You don't mean you were attacked?'

'No, it was more my fault than his.'

I liked her honesty. When I examined her I found a small spurting vulval artery which was controlled in due course by a small pack with external counter-pressure.

As I turned into the gates of my own house a man appeared out of the darkness and followed me down the drive. It was Bob Stanford.

'Will she be alright?' he asked.

'Yes, I think so, Bob. Are you — she's not a relative or anything?'

'No, it was me.'

'I see.' The shock lasted a second or so. 'Well, she should be quite alright as far as the injury is concerned.' I felt disgusted and drove the car on into the garage. There I sat for several minutes thinking. Such behaviour was rare in those days and it was out of character.

I never thought of myself as a prude but I found this difficult to forgive. Why should Bob Stanford, a man with an unusually attractive wife, risk an adventure like this? He might easily have made her pregnant and this would certainly have ruined his marriage. His wife was presumably at home looking after the baby, while he was out philandering with a girl of nineteen. The more I thought about it the more harshly I condemned him.

In medical practice one makes contact with these small

dramas only at odd points. I had no idea what had led Bob into this affair but as usual it was the woman in the case — his wife — who told me more about it in due course.

Bridget came to see me some weeks later looking the picture of misery. She wanted to talk and I let her. The event was far more unusual in those days than now, and it seemed likely to shatter their happiness for a long time to come. It had only happened once and apparently Bob was full of remorse. My inclination was to join in the condemnation of her husband but this wouldn't help anyone.

Proceeding on the lines of trying to help each one of a couple under strain to understand the other, I tried to act as counsel for the defence. I did my best, but as I heartily blamed Bob in my own mind I doubt if I was very convincing. I pointed out that he was a vigorous man who had probably suffered even more than she had over the baby's illness, that to be unemployed and at home nursing a sick child would be to him the depths of effeminacy. He was an attractive man and had probably been tempted by the girl and so on. This was the best I could do but I failed dismally. I discovered that she had refused to sleep with Bob for weeks so I redoubled my efforts.

'He told you about it himself?' I asked.

'I got it out of him when he came home late.'

'He didn't deny it?'

'No, he couldn't.'

I didn't support his behaviour but I couldn't help some admiration at the way Bob had waited to be sure the other girl was alright before he went home. If he hadn't, he would have been home earlier and Bridget might never have 'got it out of him' as she said.

'He waited to see me to make sure the girl was alright, you know,' I pointed out. 'That was what made him late.' Hardly a mitigating circumstance but I could think of nothing better.

'Yes, he told me.'

'Some men would have denied it,' I said. 'He was honest. He's been through a bad time with being laid off. So have you, I know, but you've got to forget it. You've got a good man there, Bridget. Don't throw him away.'

'It's him that's thrown me away.'

I had no idea how my words had been taken and could only guess over the months that followed. There was no question of the marriage breaking down, although in those days adultery was the one accepted reason for divorce. Divorce didn't happen in the working classes. Who knows what might happen today if Bridget had met half a dozen of her friends who wanted to welcome her into the league of divorcees.

It was about three months later that she came to see me again. She was pregnant. Bob had found work at one of the factories and she was very happy.

After I had examined her she spoke about their recent quarrel and it was then that she opened my eyes.

'You talked about Bob being miserable because he was out of work,' she said. 'Well, it *was* that in a way, but it was more than that. We were both wretched because he was on the dole but do you know what I found out when we kept talking about it? His going with that girl made him feel somehow better, successful, if you know what I mean. He thought he was no good for anything, but when that girl fell for him he felt he wasn't down and out after all. I'm sure that was it. If he hadn't been feeling so useless it would never have happened. Can you understand what I mean?'

'Yes, I can,' I said. 'I certainly can.' And when I thought about it, this seemed to me a profoundly wise and very generous piece of understanding on her part. I wished very much that this piece of sound sense had occurred to me first. My eyes had been opened by the very patient I was meant to be advising.

Looking back from this distance, I see Bob's action as a parallel with the acts of violence and vandalism of the unemployed in the eighties. The need seems to be a degree of self-assertion which breaks the accepted codes of behaviour. Adultery was violence enough in 1931. It wouldn't be now.

A few months later their son Jack was born. Bob did well in the factory and the family fortunes improved. He was in the army during the war and got three stripes, coming home safely in 1946.

The next episode in the family occurred in 1950. Their son Jack had done well at school, and had achieved high enough marks in what are now called A levels to ensure a place at university. He had then got his first choice and a place at Cambridge.

At that time Somerset County Council was far from generous in its grants for higher education, but Jack Stanford was an exceptional case and he was given the maximum grant. All was well and the future couldn't be brighter for a family I had become very much attached to — until one day in July 1950 when Bob came to see me.

'You're not going to believe this, Dr Lane,' he said. 'It's our Jack.'

'Yes?' I waited while Bob showed signs of agitation which made me wonder what on earth was coming. He wasn't anxious, but furious, so it wouldn't be a matter of illness but probably some misdemeanour. If Jack had broken into Buckingham Palace, Bob couldn't have looked more distressed.

'There's a young girl called Mandy Blacket and she's got herself pregnant. She says it's our Jack and he doesn't deny it.'

Mandy Blacket was the girl I wrote about in my earlier diary. The daughter of a notorious 'non-payer', she had at the age of six found me so attractive that she insisted on walking with me to my car whenever I visited their house. She also insisted on holding my hand, and as her hands were always sticky with jam or treacle or other messy substance, I was left with one hand in need of an urgent wash before I could decently visit another house. I always intended to keep a pair of anti-sticky gloves in the car for self-defence but of course I never remembered. There was something rather attractive about the child in spite of her infuriating habits, and in the next fifteen years she grew into a veritable sex symbol in the place.

The full horror of the situation dawned on me slowly. In those days a young man who made a girl pregnant was still expected to marry her instead of blaming her for not being on the pill. A family as honourable as the Stanfords would certainly fulfill their obligations but Jack's career would

227

not only be in danger, it would be ruined. A young man of eighteen who was married would never be accepted at Cambridge, and besides he would have to earn his living at once.

In a few minutes I was as flattened and distressed as Bob. I could offer no help and no hope. Bob complained bitterly.

'The blasted young fool,' he said, 'to go and ruin himself like that. He must be mad — mad. Well he'll get no help from me, I can tell you. He can try for a job at the pit. They're still taking men on now and again. And he can marry this — female and be as bloody miserable as he deserves.'

He ranted on for some time and I listened, hoping he would clear some of the fury out of his system. At last, when he stopped for lack of breath, I asked, 'What did you think I could do to help?'

'Twas Bridget. She made me come. Said you might be able to suggest something. What else could we do?'

'Don't be too hard on him, Bob. It may have been the girl's fault. You should know that well enough. You knew it in 1931, don't you remember?'

He ground his teeth. 'Tis no excuse. I were in trouble at home, on the dole, and the girl was a decent young woman, not a bloody tart. Young Jack had the world at his feet. Everything in his favour and he goes and does this.'

'I seem to remember that back in 1931 you had more generous understanding,' I said. Bob thumped my desk with his fist but said nothing.

I thought for a moment, and the sheer injustice of the affair made me almost as angry as Bob. 'Well I'll tell you what I'd do, Bob. I wouldn't let him marry her unless he really wants to. There's no sense in making himself and the girl miserable for the rest of their lives. If there's maintenance money to be paid you'll have to advance it yourself, and let Jack pay it back when he's earning. He's got the chance to earn more than you've ever done. What about that?'

I felt I was being bold and almost wicked, although

from this distance my suggestion seems far from out-rageous. But then, traditions have changed.

Bob was shocked at first and then interested. 'Twouldn't be right,' he said. 'The young fool.'

'How long had they been carrying on?' I asked.

'There was nothing like that. It happened one night after a dance. You see, young Jack's finished with his schooling and just waiting for the university. He's doing a labouring job, temporary like. Not enough to occupy his mind.'

'Why did you call Mandy Blacket a tart?'

'She'm always out with the boys. Everyone knows her.'

'Then how do you know Jack's the father of the baby?'

Bob stared at me. 'Jesus,' he said, 'I never thought of that. That makes it all the worse.' His mind ran swiftly over the possibilities and he added, 'Oh my God.' Then he was silent.

'I think in this case, Bob, you'll have to stop him promising to marry the girl. At least while you have time to think about it. Not to marry the girl would be the lesser of two evils. He must go on with his career whatever happens. You can't be sure he was responsible for the girl's pregnancy anyway.'

'She'll say so and Jack don't deny it, so what can you do? She knows a good lad when she sees one, blast her.'

'There's no hurry. Don't decide anything. Whatever you do, don't let Jack make any promises. Let's wait a bit.'

We talked round the subject for a while and then he left, both of us in low spirits. When I think of the number of patients' troubles I have shared, I am surprised at my continued good health!

I felt uneasy at the advice I had given and expected to be strongly criticised by Jessica. After surgery I spoke to Tom Wyburn about the affair and his condemnation was whole-hearted.

'It's this appalling lack of moral standards, Lane,' he said. 'As I see it, if the boy has been fool enough to make a girl pregnant he'll have to pay the price.'

'But what a price! Ruin, plain and simple. And he may not be the father.'

'Is the girl likely to admit that?'

229

'I doubt it. You'd say they ought to marry?'

'I see no alternative in an honourable family.'

My unease increased.

That evening, of course, Jessica had the whole story and to my great relief she agreed with me utterly.

'What sort of girl is she?' she asked.

'Blousy, attractive in a way, full-lipped and full-breasted, shapely. Bob Stanford called her a tart. He said everyone knows her character. I have no idea whether she is really promiscuous.'

'You can find that out when you see her, but you don't even know yet whether she is pregnant, do you?'

'That's a point. Better wait till she comes to see me — if she does.'

She came alright, with her mother. It was about the end of July. She was looking very pretty, very prim and proper and quite happy. Her last period, she said, was May 12th and she had had sex with Jack Stanford about ten days later, and had missed her June and July periods. It sounded as though there was no doubt that Jack was the father. If she had conceived about May 22nd she would have been about nine weeks pregnant.

I examined her and there was no doubt about the pregnancy. I always found it difficult to be sure about the duration of a pregnancy between six and nine weeks, but in this case it was easy. She was three months pregnant — a time when even the non-expert can be pretty sure of the dates. This would fit in with the usual spree at the time of Melbrook Fair but not with a period on May 12th. I checked the uterus again and there was no doubt about it. She was three months pregnant.

Mrs Blacket was acting as the injured mother who was kind and warm-hearted enough to forget and forgive — as soon as the marriage had been agreed. She spoke as though marriage to Jack Stanford had already been arranged. When I had completed my examination and Mandy had dressed I said to her, 'I wonder if I could talk to Mandy alone, Mrs Blacket?'

There was no reason for her to agree but she did without hesitation and went out into the waiting-room.

'Have you made any actual plans, Mandy? About getting married, I mean. Was Jack Stanford a regular boyfriend?'

'Oh, yes, we've known each other since we were kids.'

'But when did you have sex with him first?'

'Not proper sex until about two months ago.'

'Before that you were friends but no sex?'

'Well, you know, we played around a bit.'

'But no real sex?'

'Not really.'

'Until when?'

'It was after a dance. About the end of May it was.'

I did my best not to show my relief. 'And you had another boyfriend earlier on?'

'Yes, but we've broken it off.'

'And you had sex with this other boy earlier?'

'Well yes, once or twice.'

'Mandy, it's very important to marry the real father of your baby.'

'Yes, it was Jack Stanford.'

'Are you sure?'

'Of course I'm sure.'

'Did you have sex with Jack at Melbrook Fair time?'

'No.'

'With anyone else?'

'Well I might have done.'

'What does that mean? Mandy, I'm thinking about your future. If you are going to marry you must marry the father of your baby. Don't you see that? If you had sex at Melbrook Fair time, please tell me.'

'Alright, I did.'

'With someone you know well?'

'Yes.'

'Well, he is the father of your baby.'

'But I didn't fall till after that. I had my periods after that.'

'You may have bled but it wasn't a period. You have been pregnant since the end of April. You are three months now and the baby is due at the end of January. How many times did you have sex with Jack?'

231

She hesitated. 'Only the once.'

'And that was at the end of May?'

'Yes.'

'Your earlier boyfriend is the father of your baby.'

She was silent. I couldn't help liking the girl; she had probably made a genuine mistake. 'Can I talk to Mum?' she said.

'Let's have her in.' I was certain now that Jack was not the father, and if paternity was contested there was a strong case to prove it. She was certainly three months pregnant.

Mrs Blacket came in, still looking demure and injured. 'Well, Mrs Blacket,' I said, 'Mandy is three months pregnant. She conceived her baby at Melbrook Fair time and she is due at the end of January. The father is the boy she had sex with then, who I gather is her regular boyfriend. If Mandy wants to marry him I expect you'll be seeing him or his parents straight away.'

'But it wasn't her old boyfriend. It was Jack Stanford.'

'No, Mandy tells me she had sex with Jack only once, and that was the end of May. She was four weeks pregnant then so it couldn't have been him. I think it is very important if you want her to marry to go straight to the right man. You see, if you go to the wrong man and he can prove it wasn't him, you'd be in difficulties. Do you see what I mean?'

She was silent for a moment, then looked at Mandy and spoke the name of the other young man. They seemed to accept the situation and I never knew whether they had really thought Jack Stanford was the father, or whether they merely preferred him to the other boy if they could get him.

'Alright,' I said, 'she'll need to see me again in a month at the latest. Make an appointment for the antenatal clinic with Miss Jamieson as you go out, will you?'

I got up and opened the door. I didn't want to be involved in any argument and by good fortune my authoritative manner paid off.

I sighed with relief when they left the room and wrote down careful notes of the whole interview. When I had time to think about the case I wanted to call and tell the Stanfords they had no need to worry any more, but I resisted the temptation. It would have been a gross breach of confidence to tell them what Mandy had told me. I knew Mrs Blacket would take my advice. She was a shrewd woman and it was her only course.

It is impossible to tell how much influence a doctor has on people's lives, but I think small acts sometimes have an effect that far outweighs their apparent significance. Perhaps one could say that about anyone, but in medical practice the opportunities for a good or bad influence are greater.

Jack's career went ahead as planned and he became eminently successful. I never met the wife he married some years later but I was told they were a happy family.

It is tempting to end this chapter at this auspicious point, but there is another episode to the family story of the Stanfords and its ending, though superficially sad, was in fact triumphant.

Bob and Bridget had a long, stable and happy marriage. They grew old with us and had grandchildren before we did. They had great joy and pride from Jack's success but Bob, in his late sixties, developed a cancer of the lung.

Hospital had little to offer except a slight prolongation of his life and it was decided to nurse him at home. The real strain of this fell, of course, on Bridget. I urged her several times to let me get Bob into hospital but she refused.

'How long will it be?' she asked me and I had to tell her, 'About three months.'

'Well,' she replied, 'if we've only got a few months more together I want him near me. You must know what it means to be together. You'd be the same.'

To which there was no answer.

She seemed to grow weaker and thinner as Bob did, and once I asked her whether she had anything else wrong with her. 'No,' she said. 'I get a bit tired but I'm alright.'

'I think I ought to examine you,' I said to her once.

'No you won't,' she answered.

We managed to keep him fairly comfortable and after a

while I visited him daily. When the end was getting near I persuaded Bridget to let him go into the cottage hospital for terminal care. I watched her sitting holding his hand through the many hours until he died. Once I said to myself, 'When our turn comes it will be just the same. When it's the end for one of us we'll be together.' How happily, almost romantically, one can view the end of life when it seems so far away!

Bob died and after the funeral I called on Bridget. It was then that I discovered the extent of what she had been through. Her tears soon disappeared and she said, 'I can tell you now. I've got something wrong with my inside.' The story was soon told. She had been suffering from symptoms of uterine cancer for months but had kept it all to herself. It was cancer, not fatigue, that had undermined her strength.

'Why on earth didn't you tell me?' I said. 'It could probably have been quite easily treated if I had known early enough.'

'You'd have made me go into hospital for an operation and I wasn't going to leave Bob as he was then. Besides I didn't want it to drag on a long time after Bob.'

The last year of their marriage had been hard, but as it turned out her decision not to have her condition treated saved her from some years of sad widowhood. She went rapidly downhill and died less than four months after Bob.

Jessica was fond of quoting to me some lines of Browning's Rabbi Ben Ezra: —

Grow old along with me!
The best is yet to be,
The last of life for which the first was made:
Our times are in his hand
Who saith 'A whole I planned'
Youth shows but half; trust God: see all, nor be afraid.

How often I have witnessed an end of life that was very far from 'the best', which was in fact sad, lonely and painful. Browning surely didn't know what he was talking about. Yet sometimes the words are triumphantly true. If a good marriage ends on a note of achievement — and Bridget's courage was indeed an achievement — and with a short period of separation, there is something triumphant about it. But the ring of truth can only be heard by those with a faith which matches that of Robert Browning.

THE END

THE PAST IS MYSELF
by Christabel Bielenberg

'It would be difficult to overpraise this book. Mrs Bielenberg's experience was unique and her honesty, intelligence and compassion makes her account of it moving beyond words'
The Economist

Christabel Bielenberg, a niece of Lord Northcliffe, married a German lawyer in 1934. She lived through the war in Germany, as a German citizen, under the horrors of Nazi rule and Allied bombings. *The Past is Myself* is her story of that experience, an unforgettable portrait of an evil time.

'This autobiography is of exceptional distinction and importance. It deserves recognition as a magnificent contribution to international understanding and as a document of how the human spirit can triumph in the midst of evil and persecution'
The Economist

'Marvellously written'
The Observer

'Nothing but superlatives will do for this book. It tells its story magnificently and every page of its story is worth telling'
Irish Press

'Intensely moving'
Yorkshire Evening News

0 552 99065 5 £2.95

ANY FOOL CAN BE A PIG FARMER
by James Robertson

A walloping, rollicking, trotter's eye view of life as a pig farmer in North Wales.

Cats, dung, and overdrafts are the three things you can be sure of finding on every farm. But on James Robertson's farm there were also rats, bats, and a boa constrictor. And of course there were the pigs . . .

Sow Number Seven, Queen of the Pen and winner of all the porcine gang wars.

George, who was supposed to father piglets on all the tribe, but fell in love with Number Eleven and wore all the hair from her back.

Duke, whose idea of being sexy was to come galumphing up and take a jump at the sow of his choice. As he weighed the best part of a ton several promising romances were squashed until he was put on a diet.

James Robertson was kicked, bitten, piddled on, and infected with pig lice. But he survives and lives to tell the tale in *Any Fool Can Be A Pig Farmer*.

0 552 12399 4 £1.75

HOVEL IN THE HILLS
by Elizabeth West

A warm, funny, moving account of the simple life in rural Wales.

She was a typist. He was a mechanic. One day Elizabeth and Alan West did what many people spend a lifetime dreaming of doing – they took to the hills. *Hovel in the Hills* is the story of the first nine years of their new life in a semi-derelict farmhouse overlooking Snowdonia. It is a heart-warming and salutary tale that abounds with the joys, and the dilemmas, of opting out of the rat race.

'Mrs West writes in a lively, humorous, down-to-earth style . . . an absorbing account of a brave experiment'
Sunday Times

'I don't think I have read a better book of its kind . . . Mrs West writes remarkably well with just the right element of humour'
Daily Telegraph

'The best book I have read about getting away from it all'
Western Mail

'Conveys the joy in the countryside, in wild things and in coping for oneself'
The Times

0 552 10907 X   £1.50

DIARY OF A MEDICAL NOBODY
by Kenneth Lane

In 1929 Dr Kenneth Lane, newly qualified and mortgaged up to the hilt in order to buy himself into a practice, set off for a small country town in Somerset. He was to spend his medical life there and, from his beginnings as the new young doctor (whom nobody wanted to consult), was to become the much loved 'Old Doctor' . . .

His practice covered a kaleidoscope of English life . . . miners in the nearby colliery, farmworkers and gypsies in the surrounding countryside, and monks from the Abbey. He worked before penicillin, the National Health, or widespread birth control, and at a time when rival practices fought neck and neck for private patients.

A warm, wonderful book, rich with characters from rural England.

0 552 12033 2 £1.75

A SELECTED LIST OF AUTOBIOGRAPHIES
AND BIOGRAPHIES AVAILABLE FROM CORGI BOOKS

While every effort is made to keep prices low, it is sometimes necessary to increase prices at short notice. Corgi Books reserve the right to show new retail prices on covers which may differ from those previously advertised in the text or elsewhere.

The prices shown below were correct at the time of going to press.

ORDER FORM

All these books are available at your book shop or newsagent, or can be ordered direct from the publisher. Just tick the titles you want and fill in the form below.

CORGI BOOKS, Cash Sales Department, P.O. Box 11, Falmouth, Cornwall.

Please send cheque or postal order, no currency.

Please allow cost of book(s) plus the following for postage and packing:

U.K. Customers—Allow 55p for the first book, 22p for the second book and 14p for each additional book ordered, to a maximum charge of £1.75.

B.F.P.O. and Eire—Allow 55p for the first book, 22p for the second book plus 14p per copy for the next seven books, thereafter 8p per book.

Overseas Customers—Allow £1.00 for the first book and 25p per copy for each additional book.

NAME (Block Letters) ....

ADDRESS ....

....